PROFESSOR PAUL LEE

Practical Regeneration

No Hacks - Just science, systems & results

©Professor Paul Lee 2026

This First Edition published: February 2026 by FCM Publishing
978-1-917377-36-2 Paperback Edition
978-1-917377-37-9 E-book Edition

All rights reserved.

The right of Professor Paul Lee to be identified as the author of this Work has been asserted in accordance with sections 77 and 78 of the Copyright, Designs and Patents Act 1988.

No part of this publication may be reproduced, stored in a retrieval system, or transmitted in any form or by any means, electronic, mechanical, photocopying, recording or otherwise, without prior written permission from the publisher. Unauthorised distribution, scanning or uploading of this Work is prohibited.

This publication is intended to provide accurate and authoritative information regarding the subject matter covered. It is sold with the understanding that the publisher is not engaged in providing medical or other professional services. If expert assistance is required, the services of a qualified professional should be sought.

All illustrations and images remain the copyright of their respective creators and are used with permission. No infringement is intended. If you believe your copyright has been used in error, please contact the publisher so that the appropriate credit or action can be taken.

Cover Design by Danji Designs

This book is dedicated to my family.

To my wife Bethan, and to my children Morgan, Ffion, and Owen — you are my reason to keep building, questioning, and believing that youth, strength, and longevity are shaped by intention and daily choices. This book exists because of the future we share.

This book is also dedicated to the memory of my mother-in-law, Hefin Whiting.

Hefin was, in every way that mattered, a second mother to me. I knew her for over twenty-five years. She was a true Welsh lady — full of heart, kindness, and humanity. She lived by principle rather than ambition, always thinking of others first.

Her life reflects the deeper meaning of living forever. Not through time, but through legacy. Not through biology alone, but through values.

We live forever through what we pass on — strength, knowledge, kindness, and care. In that sense, Hefin lives forever, as do all those whose actions continue to shape others long after they are gone.

Contents

Introduction - Why I Had To Write This Book	1
Pillar 1 - Physics: The Structure of Healing	11
How often do you think about your body as a whole?	13
Movement Analysis and Why It Matters	20
Common Dysfunction Patterns	23
The Impact of Posture and Gravity	28
Gravity's Real Effect	32
Recognising Rhythm Loss and Compensation Patterns	36
What Your Gait Is Really Telling You	42
Simple Physics: Torque, Angles and Joint Stress	48
MAI-Motion - Motion Analysis Intelligence	54
Applying These Principles in Everyday Life	58
Tuning Into Internal Signals	64
Energy Input and the Physical Signals You Might Be Missing	71
What Is Grounding (and Why Should You Care)?	80
The effects of heat waves, sound waves and electromagnetic fields on the body	84
How Therapies Connect to Physics	87
Introducing The Regen PhD Pod	94
Chapter Summary	98
Practical Section	101
Daily Tools That Actually Help	104
Pillar 2 - Chemistry: The Invisible War	105
Medicine is chemistry in action	107
The Problem with How We See Chemistry	110
Why chemistry matters more than you think.	113
The Family Tree of Modern Medicine	117

The Modern Problem: Too Much, Too Blind	120
Your Internal MOT - Bloods, DNA and Hormones	122
Hormones - The Master Switches	129
Menopause: The Chemistry Storm	132
The Chemistry Of What You Eat	137
Advanced Chemistry - Beyond Food And Pills	146
The Science of Negative Ions	153
The Pod - Chemistry Meets Physics	156
Aromatherapy: Ancient Chemistry, Modern Science	159
What This Means for Your Future	162
The Future of Chemistry	165
Your Practical Toolkit	169
Chapter Summary	176
Pillar 3 - Biology: You Are Not a Machine	**179**
Biology – The Science of Human Living	181
What success looks like (it's boring and brilliant but no 5am club!)	185
Digestion	186
Why the Gut Leads in Biology	189
Regeneration Starts Here	193
Your Gut Talks and Your Brain Listens	198
A practical tool for gut awareness	200
Daily Tracker	201
From Theory to Action: The 14-Day Gut Reset	205
Gut Myths That Waste Time	207
Common Gut Questions	208
Practical Toolkit	210
Hormones: The Timing System of Regeneration	212
Hormones & Regeneration - The Chemical Timing System	214
Hormone Repair Readiness Check	221

Rhythms - Your Body's Timekeepers	224
Why This Matters for Regeneration	230
Regeneration Rhythm Tracker	231
Stillness - Sleep as Regeneration	234
The Nervous System	246
The Autonomic Nervous System - The Wiring You Don't Control	249
Trauma's Footprint - The Long-Term Cost	255
Regeneration Now - What Science (and Vanity) Already Offers	257
The Next Phase of Biological Regeneration	261
Practical Tools	267
Nervous System Reset Worksheet	271

Pillar 4 - Time: The Missing Variable — **277**

Time - The Hidden Force	279
The Practical Lesson	289
Practical Toolkit: REPAIR	290
Psychology of Delay	301
My Quick Guide: When Not to Wait	306
Why Monitoring Progress Keeps You From Wasting Months or Years	308
Practical Toolkit: How to Monitor Without Obsession	319
How to Value Your Health at Least as Much as Your Possessions	322
Practical Toolkit: The Health Value Audit	329
Ageing Better: Why Mindset Matters as Much as Medicine	332
How Science Is Changing the Future of Time	338
Why I engineered the Regen PhD Pod	346
Chapter Summary	348
Practical Toolkit: Working With Time	350

Habits	**353**
The Crown: The Habits of Regeneration	354
A Brief History of Habits	359
Regeneration Is A Habit	362
Designing for Success	365
Example - Designing Hydration, Not Hoping for It	369
Example - Designing Movement Into the Day	371
The 1% Rule	374
The Five-Minute Habit Arsenal	381
Regen PhD: a Toolkit designed for regeneration	387
What's Next for Regeneration	400
The Live Forever Movement	405
Acknowledgements	**407**
Author Bio	**410**
Other Books by Professor Paul Lee	**412**
Further Reading	**413**

Introduction - Why I Had To Write This Book

Over the past three years, my entire approach to medicine has changed. Once, my professional focus was on refining surgical techniques – improving hip replacements and enhancing knee procedures – pursuing marginal gains in outcomes through technical precision. It was the natural mindset of an orthopaedic surgeon embedded in a system that rewards intervention, speed and throughput.

However, that system is no longer fit for purpose. Increasingly, I began to see that patients were actively avoiding surgery. They would pursue complex and expensive alternatives, travel across the world, spend tens of thousands on new and uncommon treatments such as stem cell, all to delay or avoid being cut open. This wasn't due to ignorance or fear but a deep, intuitive understanding that surgery, while sometimes necessary, isn't always the best answer.

Within our National Health Service, the metrics of success are built around volume and conversion. In outpatient clinics, clinicians are judged not by how many patients they help but by how many they can convert to surgery. A "hit list" defines success. Ten patients seen, ten surgical bookings made – that's considered high performance. The reality, however, is that this model reduces people to numbers and symptoms, rather than individuals with complex, multifactorial health problems.

I became acutely aware that my role as a surgeon was being directed more by administrative performance indicators than by clinical judgement. Managers with no medical training judged outcomes by throughput and efficiency; little did we know, we were just creating empty wards and not following it to help people. The more surgeries booked, the more revenue generated. Meanwhile, appointment times were cut, thirty minutes became ten. Patients were rushed through assessments with no room for discussion, hesitation or context. Many weren't ready for surgery, and some didn't need it at all. No matter, the pressure to fill operating lists remained.

It became clear to me that the system was losing sight of its purpose: to care. Discussions shifted away from patient-centred treatment and towards efficiency, cost-saving and operational targets. The deeper I went, the more detached the profession became from patients, from outcomes, from ethics.

This is not a criticism of individual clinicians but of the machinery they are forced to operate within.

In that environment, I could no longer reconcile my training with my values, so I shifted direction toward a new model of regenerative care. I am still a surgeon, just one who now looks for every alternative before reaching for the scalpel. My focus is prevention, early intervention, and addressing the root cause long before the final symptom appears.

I have been awarded a PhD in Medical Engineering, a Fellowship in Regenerative Medicine and I am a Consultant Orthopaedic Surgeon. All of this allows me now to focus on regeneration.

I decided to combine my medical and engineering knowledge to provide alternative ways of helping people. After all the ethos of any medical practitioner is *Do No Harm*.

Whereas the motto of the U.S. Army Corps of Engineers is, "*Essayons*", which translates to "*Let us try!*"

Combined this speaks to me as – let's find a way to ensure that we are caring for our bodies and not placing ourselves in harm.

Cue my first book, *Regeneration by Design*. I would recommend reading it first, but it is not absolutely necessary.

From the beginning, I set out to challenge the way we think about ageing and health. Rather than waiting for problems to arise, I believe we can actively influence how well we age by understanding and supporting the body's natural regenerative abilities.

I introduced the philosophy of regenerative medicine, as a systematic, proactive approach grounded in established principles of biology, physics, chemistry and time. The four pillars as I refer to them. These four pillars represent a more

Introduction - Why I Had To Write This Book

integrated, holistic approach to health that sees the human body as a single, dynamic network.

I argued that ageing is not simply the inevitable decline of the body but a process we can influence by tipping the balance in favour of regeneration over degeneration.

Throughout the book, I explored concepts like "superhuman ageing", harnessing the body's own capacity to repair and renew. I introduced my Six Superhuman Steps: practical actions anyone can take to minimise biological stress, optimise cellular health and personalise their approach using the latest technologies, including AI.

A common example is back pain: it illustrates why prevention matters. For instance, while we routinely service our cars, most people neglect their spine until pain strikes. Yet, simple steps, like maintaining hydration, protecting joint health and understanding forces acting on the body, can make a profound difference. We understand that the right fuel, oil and water make our cars run better, although we still ignore the same principle when it comes to our bodies.

I covered the importance of cell regeneration, the role of hormones, the impact of sleep, exercise and even the healing power of a smile (don't discount this one!). I also demystified current regenerative treatments, from stem cell therapy and PRP (Platelet Rich Plasma) to the use of lasers, ultrasound, electricity and motion analysis.

One key message I emphasised is this: regeneration should not be left to chance. We can and should design for it. My background in orthopaedics and engineering has shown me that a structured, scientific approach, is what truly delivers lasting outcomes.

In short, Regeneration by Design aimed to help people take control of their health span as well as their lifespan. It laid the foundation for a regenerative life.

That book asked questions. This book answers them.

In *Regeneration by Design*, I introduced what I call the Six Superhuman Steps. These steps were never intended as a checklist or a sequence to be followed rigidly. but they form a way of thinking about the body as a system, one that must be stabilised, supported and understood before meaningful regeneration can occur.

At their core, the steps ask simple but often overlooked questions. What is disturbing the system? Are there mechanical, chemical or biological stresses preventing recovery? Are we supporting the body's natural repair processes, or constantly working against them? And crucially, are we making informed decisions early enough to change the outcome?

The framework moves from removing unnecessary disturbance, through optimising chemistry and biology, to understanding the physical forces acting on the body. It recognises that poor movement, misalignment and chronic overload are not abstract concepts but predictable contributors to degeneration. It also embraces modern tools, including digital body banking and motion analysis, not as replacements for clinical judgement, but as reference points. They give us

Introduction - Why I Had To Write This Book

something increasingly rare in medicine: a clear baseline for what "healthy" actually looks like for an individual.

Underlying all of this is time. Regeneration is not instant; delay, inaction and short-term fixes all have consequences. The decisions we make, and when we make them, often determine whether a problem resolves, stabilises or progresses toward surgery.

This book builds directly on that foundation. Rather than revisiting theory, my aim here is to show how these principles work in practice. How we assess the body, what we prioritise, which interventions matter and why. This is where regenerative medicine moves from concept to application.

This is the practical application of regenerative medicine. It is for patients, practitioners and anyone seeking a pathway out of pain, dysfunction and the surgery-first approach that dominates modern orthopaedics. It is a guide to understanding your own body, to choosing options and to reclaiming agency over your health.

Practical Regeneration is less about rejecting surgery and more about widening the options before it becomes inevitable. It is about equipping you with knowledge that the current system rarely offers and laying out a clear, structured process to assess, intervene and support true healing.

Across these chapters, I will walk through the four pillars in practice. I will explain how we test, what we look for, what interventions we use and why. I am fully aware that this approach is not going to win me many friends in surgical circles. Some of what I say may seem too far removed from traditional methods to be credible – at least at first glance. Many surgeons have been doing things a certain way for decades and see no reason to change. They've become so comfortable in the cycle of referral, injection, operation that they no longer question the long-term consequences.

Take steroid injections as an example. Routinely offered for joint pain, they are seen as low risk, convenient and cost-effective, however, they're masking the issue, rather than resolving it. Repeated use can accelerate tissue degeneration, weaken structures and delay more appropriate interventions. In the short term, they relieve pain and in the long term, they often create more problems than they solve.

This kind of short-term thinking – designed around symptoms rather than causes – is precisely what regenerative medicine seeks to move beyond.

In this next book, I want to take these ideas further and show you how to move beyond the theoretical, into practical strategies that can transform how you live every day.

The future of medicine must move beyond reactive models and into proactive, regenerative ones. We must stop asking, *"What can we cut out?"* and start asking, *"What can we restore?"* or *"How can we prevent the need?"*

This book is a small but necessary step in that direction.

"Design is a journey of discovery." - Alvin Huang

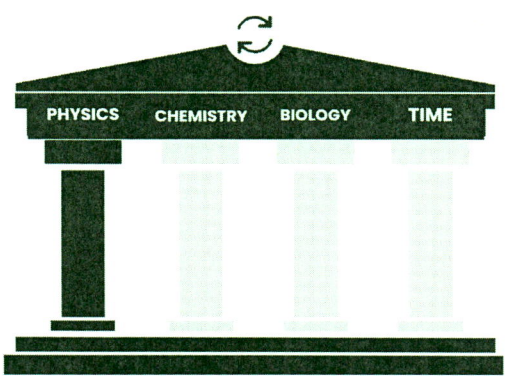

Pillar 1 - Physics:
The Structure of Healing

*"If you don't understand force and function,
you'll never fix the frame."*

Measure what can be measured, and make measureable what cannot be measured.

Galileo Galilei

How often do you think about your body as a whole?

Most people only think about bits of their body when something hurts. When your back is sore your focus goes there, the same if you have tight hamstrings and if you get a headache then it's easy just to reach for a painkiller. What you don't think is: *"Could that headache be tension in my neck? A jaw issue? Even stomach problems?"* Yes it could be. Everything is connected.

Before we get into the four pillars, I want you to pause and actually think about this: there is no single part of your body that isn't linked to something else. The body operates as a system rather than a collection of interchangeable spare parts, and while the word "holistic" technically gets close to what I mean, it has been so overused by the wellness industry that it no longer carries the strength that I want to convey. *Systemic* is the better fit because it reflects the reality of how the body works: as a single, interconnected network in which every process influences the next, rather than a set of random pieces that can be treated in isolation.

Pillar 1 - Physics: The Structure of Healing

This isn't just common sense; it's an engineering principle. In engineering school, there's a discipline called systems engineering. It's about looking at the whole system, not just isolated parts. If you only ever fix the visible fault, you never solve the root cause. The body works the same way.

Some of you are thinking: *"But Prof, my body IS made of individual parts."* Sure. Here's the truth: they don't work in isolation. Think of a car. If your tyre wears on one edge, you don't just swap the tyre and keep driving, you check the alignment and the steering. If the tracking's out, the car keeps pulling and the wear keeps coming. Your body is the same. One broken toe can mess with your knee, your hip, your spine. Not overnight but over time the pattern will show. Even a week of limping is enough to throw off your rhythm.

> **Here's a real-life example:**
>
> "I have severe arthritis in many places in my body. I was recommended to try shockwave therapy. They reviewed my entire frame and found one leg slightly shorter than the other. My hips, sacral joint, knees and ankles were all out of alignment. All of this traced back to long-standing lower back problems. For 30 years I'd carried myself wrongly and it had effectively bent the chassis of my body. I had no idea until someone pointed out how favouring one side had caused more wear, more imbalance and poor posture." - T. Mortimer

That's the point: compensation is clever until it becomes chronic. At that point it becomes the new normal, because it happens so slowly, you won't even notice it until it is too late. Overloading one spot means something else is working overtime. Do that for long enough and you don't just get pain; you get a cascade of problems. Have you ever had pain show up out of "nowhere" and thought, *"Where did that come from?"* It didn't come from "nowhere". It came from months or years of subtle misalignment, overcompensating in silence until the system said, *"Enough."*

Here's the good news: it's not too late but you have to see the problem first. You can't fix what you don't measure. The problem isn't always obvious; it often hides behind habits you've had for years. If you keep looking at each joint in isolation, you'll keep chasing symptoms instead of fixing the system.

That's why I wrote this book: to help you understand that everything is related. Energy, structure and motion are the framework of your body. When you alter physics, you can change chemistry and influence biology. That means we can often heal by improving movement, without always reaching for drugs or invasive fixes. Understand these principles and you reclaim far more control: you can handle pain more effectively, protect yourself from long-term disability and live with a noticeably higher quality of life. Your length of life may stay the same, but the experience of living it will be better.

Most people can picture muscles, joints and posture but, underneath all of that is physics. It's all about force: where it goes, where it leaks and how your body deals with it. Every movement you make, every load your body absorbs or deflects, every signal firing through your nervous system, all of it obeys the laws of physics. If you want to regenerate, you have to start with how you move, how you absorb shock, how you stand, sit, lift, bend, run, recover.

You can't fix what you don't measure.

A 1% error repeated daily is compound damage. A 1% improvement repeated daily is regeneration.

I've replaced hips that failed early through years of unmanaged force rather than age or disease. No single trauma caused it; the mechanics were just slightly off and repeated thousands of times. I've seen tendons fray the same way, tiny failures building until the whole system gives way. These are patterns, not accidents.

"We don't have the tools that can be used to easily monitor movements, so I designed them."

That's what led me to build Musculoskeletal AI Motion (MAI-Motion). It's a digital tool that measures how your body moves using only your smartphone. Why? Because the way we assess movement is broken. Most traditional assessments rely on a practitioner's eye, their angle, their attention span. You're basically at the mercy of someone's Tuesday mood. I wanted something objective, something anyone could use without a lab. MAI-Motion captures how your body loads, balances and compensates. It watches movement frame by frame and gives real, readable feedback, removing guesswork, and in return it gives you a way to see what's really going on.

You don't need high-end tech to start seeing; you need awareness, because the signs are already there, and you simply haven't tuned into them yet.

That's what this chapter gives you. It shows you how to observe your own body. If your shoes wear unevenly, that's pressure data. If your knee hurts only on stairs, that's a force signal. If your spine twists every time you reach for the kettle, that's daily torque being dumped into the wrong joint. These signals tell the story before the pain does.

We'll also cover the simple tools that build better mechanics – wobble boards, standing desks, mirror checks, step drills – to help you train awareness, build rhythm and restore symmetry. Motion isn't random. It's a pattern and patterns can be corrected.

MAI-Motion adds depth to this process. With just your phone, you can capture movement and get real feedback that is objective pattern recognition. Motion fingerprints - no two people move in the same way.

MAI-Motion is built around the **C.R.A.F.T. system**, five key markers of movement health:
- **Control** - Can you manage your joints deliberately? Wobbles, rigid movements, hesitation tell us control is slipping.
- **Repeatability** - Do you move the same way every time? If not, your body is compensating or unstable.
- **Asymmetry** - Do both sides move equally? One arm swinging higher, one leg landing harder.

Pillar 1 - Physics: The Structure of Healing

- **Flow** - Are your transitions smooth? Flow shows whether your system is integrated or fighting itself.
- **Twist** - Are you rotating through areas that should stay stable? Spinal twists during gait or uneven loading add up to strain.

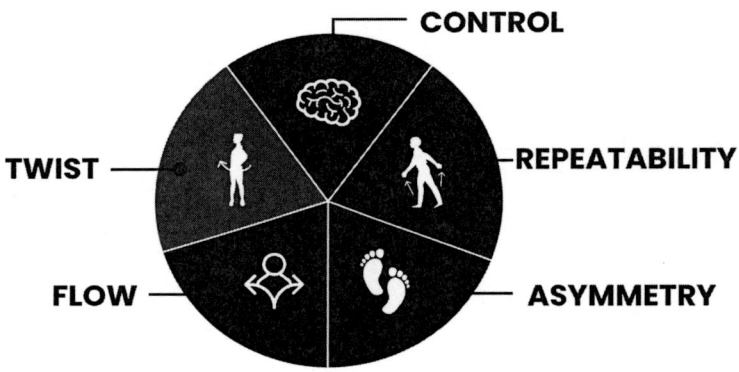

Ask yourself: are you controlling your movement, or bracing your way through it? Are you consistent, or adjusting mid-task? Do both sides behave the same? Is there flow, or is the system patching holes?

At the end of this chapter, I'll show you how to download MAI-Motion and use it yourself. But whether you use tech or not, the goal is the same: see more, know more and intervene earlier. Your body is always giving you feedback, you just need to learn how to read it.

In the sections ahead, we'll break down:
- How to observe and interpret your movement
- The impact of posture and gravity
- Recognising rhythm loss and compensation patterns
- What your gait is really telling you

- Simple physics: torque, angles, joint stress
- How energy inputs affect recovery and movement
- The role of sound, heat, light and magnetic fields on repair

Most importantly, you'll learn how to respond, rather than reacting, so your body regenerates on purpose, not just by luck or time. Let's build that from the ground up.

Movement Analysis and Why It Matters

How you walk, sit, or get up from a chair isn't just habit, it's data. What we're doing is making the invisible visible. It shows where you're compensating, how your body is balancing load and where injury is building before you feel it.

You can begin right now. Watch yourself walk past a shop window. Does one shoulder dip? Do your feet flare out? Film yourself standing up from a chair. Is one knee doing more work? These are patterns.

If you're concerned about how you walk or have pain in your knees, hips, or back, consider getting a foot scan. This will give you a real-time map of force: a foot scan shows how your feet absorb load and whether you're carrying imbalance without realising it. You stand or walk on a pressure plate or mat while sensors measure how force travels through your feet. It can reveal if you're overloading the inside or outside edge, if your arches are collapsing, or if you're shifting weight unevenly from left to right.

Why does that matter? The foot is the foundation for everything above it. If you're compensating in your stance or stride, that load travels into your knees, hips and spine. We see people with hip pain whose scans show they've been favouring one leg for years. Or with back pain that traces to an ankle problem. A foot scan lets you catch these patterns early, before pain leads to damage.

When you know what to look for, you start to feel where your motion is leaking energy or building stress. Once you see the pattern, you can change the outcome, that way you can train and protect, and because it's tracked over time, you can see your improvement. You're not relying on pain anymore, you're using data**.** That's where regeneration begins, with measurement and action.

Begin with something simple, such as filming yourself walking for ten seconds. Repeat this once a week and compare the footage. Look for changes in rhythm, stability and ease. You might notice a steadier stride, a more balanced hip line or a smoother transition from step to step. These subtle shifts are genuine signs of progress. The aim is steady improvement that protects your body over time. When you act early and pay attention to these small details, you give your system the conditions it needs for long-term regeneration and resilience.

Movement falls into three categories:
- **Daily:** Walking, sitting, getting out of bed, reaching for the cupboard
- **Functional**: Carrying shopping bags, picking up your child, cleaning, dog-walking
- **Athletic:** Gym sessions, running, cycling, competitive sport

Pillar 1 - Physics: The Structure of Healing

Each one places different demands on the body. Sit for eight hours and you build a different set of compensations than someone who stacks shelves for eight hours. Prolonged sitting tightens the hips, weakens the glutes and changes the curvature of the spine, whilst physical labour often builds uneven strength – one side dominant, rotation through the lower back, load on one knee.

No movement is neutral; every habit reinforces a pattern.
You remember that childhood song:
The leg bone's connected to the knee bone,
The knee bone's connected to the thigh bone,
The thigh bone's connected to the hip bone.

Biomechanically and medically speaking the song is wrong but the point is true. If one joint is out of alignment, it affects everything above and below. Think of it like dominoes – tip one and the rest start falling, or worse, they fall unevenly.

Common Dysfunction Patterns

- Foot flare: One or both feet angle outwards. Often driven by tight hips or weak external rotators. Long-term: alters knee tracking, contributes to hip stress.
- Hip drop: When one side of the pelvis dips while walking. Suggests glute medius weakness. Long-term: imbalance in spinal load, lower back pain.
- Shoulder hike: Chronic tension or compensation on one side. May come from repetitive bag-carrying or poor desk ergonomics.
- Pelvic tilt: Anterior tilt compresses the lumbar spine and shortens the front hip structures. Common in desk-based workers.

None of these patterns arrive with a warning sign. They sneak in slowly, like bad habits do.

Here's a real-life example

Raj, a 38-year-old postman. No major injury history but nagging knee pain. On video analysis, we saw a consistent foot flare on the left, hip drop on the right and minimal glute engagement. Over a 12-hour shift, these mechanics repeated thousands of times. A simple retraining plan: foot drills, hip stability work and glute reactivation, led to significant improvement within six weeks.

Raj didn't need surgery, just new habits. He now moves so well he says the stairs at work feel shorter. They're not but his knees believe it.

This is what MAI-Motion helps make objective. With just a short video, the system analyses your movement through the C.R.A.F.T. lens. When you see how you move, you can start to shift it.

Warning Signs

Early red flags are easy to ignore:
- Clicking joints that persist.
- One-sided tightness that repeats.
- Slower leg lift on one side.
- Needing momentum to get up from a chair.
- Swaying when brushing your teeth.

They're your body's version of "fix this before I really get your attention".

Regen tips:

Building Self-Awareness

Use mirrors. Use your phone. More importantly, use your attention.

- Stand in front of a mirror and note shoulder height.
- Film yourself from the front and side while walking. Yes, it feels weird. So does limping for 20 years.
- Try balancing on one leg. Is one easier?
- Sit down and stand up – is one leg doing more work?

Make a checklist:

- Do I feel tighter on one side?
- Are my shoes wearing unevenly?
- Do I lean on one elbow while working?
- Do I avoid turning one way?

Start a movement diary. Weekly notes. Short clips. One line of observation. "Right shoulder higher today." "Felt stiff getting up." "Hip clicks on stairs." It might not be a New York Times Bestseller but your future self will thank you.

Movement Myth

"Just move more" gets said a lot but if the movement's poor, more of it only reinforces the damage. Just moving more with poor habits increases wear. It teaches the wrong pattern and pushes already strained joints harder.

Strategic movement matters. Think reps with awareness, not reps for the sake of reps.

Micro-Practices

Change happens in small, repeated acts.
- Brush your teeth while standing on one leg. If it feels strange, good. Strange means your brain is paying attention.
- Squat to pick things up instead of bending.
- Set a timer to shoulder roll every hour.
- Alternate foot leads on the stairs.
- Stand up and sit down without using your hands.
- Do one-minute wall sits during coffee breaks.

I have a client who has alarms on her phone for almost all of these activities. It does make for interesting meetings, and her phone is constantly bleeping but she is considerably healthier than she was 18 months ago before she started setting the alarms. This may not be practical for you but there are apps that can remind you to stand and walk around when you've been sitting at your desk for too long. For others it is just a case of reminding themselves to think before they start any activity.

Each micro-practice is a signal, a step towards long-term joint protection. That's physics in real life: load, angles, wear. It adds up, or it breaks down.

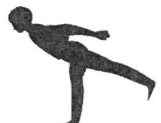

ONE-LEG BALANCE WHILE BRUSHING TEETH

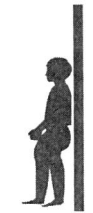

WALL SIT AGAINST A WALL.

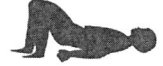

GLUTE BRIDGE LYING ON THE FLOOR.

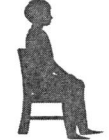

TOE TAPS WHILE SEATED

The Impact of Posture and Gravity

Posture Under Load

The reason posture matters in a book about regeneration is simple: alignment determines how efficiently your tissues repair. When force travels through the body cleanly, cells can use their energy for healing rather than constant compensating. Regeneration begins with how you carry load in everyday life.

We don't often think about gravity; it's something we take for granted and that happens to us. However, gravity is working on you constantly, while you walk, lift, carry bags, even queue for coffee. If your joints are not stacked properly, strain multiplies fast. Good posture spreads load evenly. poor posture dumps it in weak spots.

For instance, someone with flat feet loses natural shock absorption. Knees and hips step in to carry that extra load. Over time, we see the problems cascade: arches collapse, knees rotate inwards, pelvis tilts, back pain follows. One fault starts the pattern. That is why we call this systems thinking: small errors compound over time.

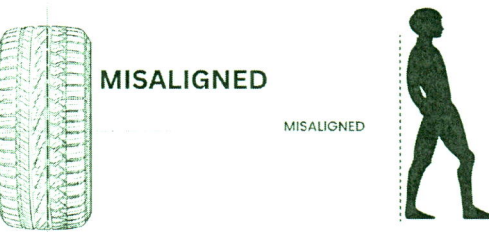

When this cascade continues unchecked, the tissues spend more time protecting than repairing, which slows recovery and accelerates wear. Restoring alignment restores the conditions that allow regeneration to happen more easily.

Your posture is how you respond to gravity's constant force. Either your structure absorbs the load well, or something compensates and when compensation runs the show long enough, problems start.

Posture is more than standing rigid like you are on parade. It is about balance and load management. Is your head stacked over your spine? Are your hips sitting over your knees and ankles? Or is something off? When the head shifts forwards, gravity increases the load through the neck, and when one hip settles lower than the other, the spine adjusts to keep balance. These changes seem small, but they quietly redirect force into areas that were never meant to carry it for long.

Think of posture as scaffolding. If one strut is out, the whole frame carries stress in the wrong places. Physics shapes every structure in the body and alignment works best when the system is balanced rather than overstretched.

Here's a real-life example

James is 42, works in finance and spends 10 hours a day at a desk. Over the past year, he started noticing tightness in his right shoulder and occasional tingling in his hand. His GP sent him to a physio, who treated the shoulder. The pain eased, then came back.

What no one had checked was his posture. When James was filmed at his desk, it was obvious: he leaned heavily on his right elbow, dropped his right shoulder and rotated his neck slightly left all day. That small misalignment, multiplied across thousands of hours, changed muscle tension, compressed nerves and created pain.

He fixed it by adjusting his desk, adding two posture resets a day and setting reminders for micro-breaks. Within three weeks, the symptoms eased. James said the fix was so simple he felt cheated out of all the stretching he had been doing. Once his posture improved, his body had the space to recover instead of constantly compensating.

As you can see, posture can be improved without endless doctor appointments; what you need is awareness and small, consistent actions.

Start with a mirror check. Side view: can you line up ear, shoulder, hip and ankle? Don't force it, just notice. Awareness always comes first.

Next, try a reset drill. Stand with your back against a wall: heels, bum, shoulder blades and head touching the wall. Hold for 30 seconds a day. That simple habit retrains your sense of neutral position.

Remember: posture is not static.
>
> Walking is posture in motion
> Sitting is posture under pressure
> Lifting is posture under load.

When you start to see posture as a moving system, you realise how tiny habits create big changes for better or worse.

Regen tips:

A standing desk or laptop riser helps restore natural alignment through the spine and hips, which reduces the strain that builds during long periods of sitting. It keeps the body moving between positions rather than collapsing into a single shape for hours at a time.

Or alternatively

Sitting on a Pilates ball for short periods activates the deep postural muscles that support your spine, strengthens the body's natural stabilisers and encourages subtle movement, rather than the fixed compressed positions that create stiffness and fatigue

Gravity's Real Effect

Gravitational loading is the silent stressor: every day, it compresses your spine, hips, knees and feet. The more out of alignment you are, the more stress your system absorbs. Standing poorly does not just look bad; it changes how force travels through your body.

Picture this: every inch your head moves forward from neutral adds roughly 5kg of load to your cervical spine. That is like asking your neck to carry a bowling ball all day long. Over time, that extra force compresses discs, irritates nerves and even alters breathing mechanics as well as the fatigue on your muscles.

For those at higher risk of bone loss, especially postmenopausal women, posture issues are more than sore muscles, they can start a chain reaction toward structural failure. This is where scanning becomes invaluable.

Professor Paul Lee

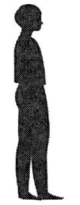
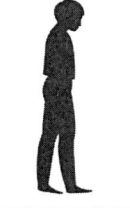

NEUTRAL   5KG LOAD PER INCH FORWARD

Bone Health Check: Why It Matters

A bone density scan (DEXA) uses low-level X-rays to measure bone mineral content and gives you a T-score comparing your bones to a healthy adult. It is simple, painless and gives a snapshot of your structural resilience.

An REM scan goes further. It includes everything DEXA offers and adds a fragility score. That score predicts how vulnerable your bones are to fracture under stress. If your score is high-risk, you should not wait for a break, you need to act now. That might include resistance training, nutrition tweaks, or supervised loading drills to protect your skeleton before it fails.

Knowing your baseline gives you clarity. It shows you exactly what your body needs so every choice you make supports the whole structure, not just the muscles on the surface.

Practical Steps
- Walk barefoot at home to build intrinsic foot strength.
- Use a foot roller for 60 seconds a day to release tension and restore arch mobility.
- Stretch calves after sitting for long periods because they take the brunt when feet fail.

- Add bone-strength drills like controlled heel slams. The micro-impact stimulates bone density, especially in the hips and spine. Do these in moderation: 10 to 15 controlled reps, three times a week. Consistency matters more than intensity.

These inputs are tiny, but physics loves consistency. Small loads, repeated often, create adaptation.

What Stairs Reveal

Stairs expose weaknesses not always noticeable on level ground, because they amplify load and coordination, making any imbalance harder to hide. Climbing stairs means fighting gravity while shifting weight forwards again and again. Doing it with poor form, leaning forwards, knees collapsing inwards and shoulders rounding multiplies joint stress.

Many people only feel knee pain on stairs, in part due to how stairs magnify inefficiencies, but they are a diagnostic goldmine if you pay attention. Clicking or sharp pain? That is the joint telling you alignment is off.

Descending stairs adds another layer: control. Muscles work eccentrically, lengthening under load to slow your descent. If your quads or glutes cannot control it, your knees take the punishment.

Here is a reality check: everyone says take the stairs for fitness. In general, yes, movement is good but bad mechanics make stairs an injury accelerator. It's better to walk on flat ground with good form than pound up and down stairs with bad form.

Next time you take the stairs, observe: does one foot always lead? Do your knees cave in? Do your feet flare? Film yourself if you can. Yes, it feels odd, but you will learn more from 10 seconds of video than 10 years of ignoring signals.

Key Takeaway - Better alignment does more than reduce strain in the moment. It frees your body to recover between movements instead of constantly managing imbalance. That shift is the foundation of regeneration: restoring the environment your body needs to renew itself every day.

Recognising Rhythm Loss and Compensation Patterns

When I talk about rhythm, I mean the natural flow of movement the body prefers: smooth timing, steady coordination and an even transfer of force from one joint to the next. When that rhythm slips, the body keeps you moving but it does it by shifting work elsewhere. That shift is compensation. A muscle that should be active fades out, another steps in and the pattern holds together for a while. Over time, those substitutions place more load on areas that were never meant to carry it and that is when strain builds quietly in the background.

Rhythm is the body's internal metronome. When it's working, you barely notice it and yet when it's off, everything feels harder, even if you can't name why. It shows up in your walk, your reach, how you step out of a car or lift a kettle. This is why a smooth rhythm means muscles are firing in the right order, joints are aligned and energy is being transferred efficiently. When rhythm falters, efficiency vanishes and wear begins

Compensation might look like a shoulder hike every time you reach overhead, or a subtle limp that shifts load to the opposite leg. You might feel tightness in your neck when the real issue is a stiff mid-back, or knee pain that starts with a locked ankle.

Here's a real-life example

Lisa, a 37-year-old yoga instructor, arrived confused by a recurring discomfort in her right hip. Her scans were clear, her flexibility was outstanding and her technique looked effortless, yet the sensation returned every time she increased her training. When we looked beyond the individual joint and examined how her whole system moved, the real picture emerged.

Motion analysis revealed what her eye couldn't catch. During lunges and turns she shifted her weight earlier than she realised, subtly unloading her right glute every time she moved through that side. The explanation for this came from her past rather than her present. Years earlier she had sprained the same ankle and never rebuilt its stability so that single weak link had been shaping her entire chain ever since. The hip was absorbing load the ankle could no longer manage.

Her yoga background gave her exceptional range, however range without control can create a false sense of security. It is a little like admiring the sweep of a suspension bridge without noticing that some of the support cables have slackened; everything looks beautiful until genuine force arrives. Her practice had masked the imbalance for years because flexibility let her compensate smoothly.

The solution wasn't dramatic. It meant returning to fundamentals, restoring ankle function, re-engaging the glutes and bringing symmetry back into her gait. After several weeks of deliberate, targeted work, her rhythm improved, her load distribution evened out and most importantly, the pain went away.

Why Rhythm Matters

When a compensation becomes routine, it directs force down the same path again and again and that repeated pathway eventually leaves its mark.

Long-term rhythm breakdown has real consequences:
- Early joint wear and osteoarthritis
- Increased risk of falls, especially in older adults
- Chronic muscle tightness and tension headaches
- Poor coordination and energy inefficiency

Think of it like this: when an orchestra plays in time, it sounds effortless. When one section drifts, the rest scramble to recover and eventually the whole thing falls apart. Your movement works the same way.

Why Rhythm Breaks

Common causes include:
- Fatigue and overtraining
- Sedentary lifestyles
- Previous injuries that weren't fully rehabilitated
- Poorly fitted footwear
- Neurological conditions affecting balance or coordination

Environmental factors matter too. Hard floors can fatigue your joints and uneven terrain demands more muscle engagement. Even how you hold your phone when walking changes your rhythm.

Your rhythm is guided by your senses: your vision, your inner ear's sense of balance and the feedback your joints give you about position and movement.

Here's a quick test: Stand on one leg with your eyes closed. Then repeat with the other leg. One side usually finds its footing; the other reminds you why the system prefers teamwork. That's giving you rhythm data.

Regen tips:

A foam roller or massage ball helps release tight areas within the muscles, restoring smoother movement and allowing the body to maintain rhythm rather than working around restrictions that build during daily life.

Common Compensation Patterns

Here's what to look for:
- Arm swing suppression: One arm doesn't swing freely, often through protective behaviour or tension. Why it matters: arm swing balances your stride; lose it and the opposite leg works overtime.

- Hip hitching: Lifting one side of the pelvis to advance the leg. A sign of glute weakness or stiff ankles. Adds lateral force through the spine and knee.
- Head bobbing: Extra bounce means the core isn't stable, so the head acts as a counterweight.
- Trunk twisting: Over-rotation when hips or core can't stabilise.
- Foot slap: Loud landings indicate poor dorsiflexion control, reducing shock absorption and hammering joints up the chain.
- Shoulder hike or roll: Over-recruitment of traps, leading to headaches and neck tension.

These patterns don't always hurt at first, but they always cost energy and, over time, cause damage. Micro-failure leads to macro-problems, every time.

What to Do About It

To course correct, these micro-practices will help:
- Walk backwards slowly for 2 minutes a day. It reboots coordination.
- Try barefoot balance work on carpet or grass.
- Pair deep, controlled breathing with movement (inhale on reach, exhale on return).

Gentle movement practices like Tai Chi also strengthen rhythm. The slow pace highlights how load shifts across the joints and trains the body to coordinate with greater control.

Introduce a movement reset: three minutes a day of rhythm restoration. March on the spot. Do slow shoulder rolls, neck tilts and hip circles. Keep it simple, consistent and body-aware.

Start building rhythm awareness by integrating short movement audits into your day. Pick a time – after brushing your teeth or before lunch – and run through a 30-second movement scan: walk, squat, reach and twist and film it once a week for feedback.

As mentioned in the last section, a movement diary helps. Track what you feel, where pain spikes and where tension builds. Patterns will appear.

And beware false positives. Some people look fluid but hide instability; flexibility isn't necessarily control.

A consistent rhythm in movement creates a predictable environment for the body. Joints load more evenly, muscles work in balance and the nervous system no longer has to firefight instability. Over time, this steady pattern preserves the structures that keep you mobile, which is the essence of regeneration.

What Your Gait Is Really Telling You

Your gait is the way your body moves through space step after step. It reveals how your joints align, how muscles coordinate and how your nervous system manages load without conscious effort. When you know how to read it, gait shows you where stress is accumulating, where efficiency is slipping and where future injury might begin.

Gait is different from general movement because it is patterned and repetitive. You can concentrate and perform a single movement well, however when you take thousands of steps a day, the body shows its true habits. That repetition magnifies small errors. A subtle hitch or slight restriction becomes a constant stress signal that tells you exactly where the system is working too hard.

Each stride has two phases: stance and swing. Stance includes heel strike, mid stance and toe off. Swing involves clearing the foot and preparing to land again. Any disruption to these phases changes how load travels through the body. Poor clearance suggests weakness or coordination issues. A heavy heel strike tells you shock absorption is failing whereas an early toe off indicates the hip is not extending properly.

Good gait also depends on sensory awareness. Your body needs an accurate sense of where each limb is in space. Poor vision, ear imbalance, fatigue, or a stiff joint can alter the information the brain receives, and this affects how you walk. When that feedback is inaccurate, your system compensates in ways that increase energy cost and reduce efficiency.

Because the body works as a chain, small deviations do not stay small. A restricted ankle alters knee mechanics, the hip adjusts and the spine shifts to keep balance. Over time, this becomes a pattern that spreads through the body. Old injuries cand play a part too - a sprained ankle from years ago can still influence how you load a knee today.

Kinetic energy also plays a role in how gait influences the rest of the body. Every step generates energy that travels upwards through the foot, knee, hip and spine. When your mechanics are clean, that energy moves smoothly through the chain and walking feels lighter and more natural. When a joint is stiff or a pattern is slightly off, that energy redirects into tissues that were never meant to handle it, which increases fatigue, reduces efficiency and gradually shapes how the body feels at the end of each day.

This is why gait and general movement don't always match. Someone can move well during a controlled task, yet their natural walking pattern tells a different story. Gait analysis reveals how the body behaves when attention is not involved and that is often where problems begin.

Simple Ways to Observe Your Gait

You can learn a lot with a short self-check. Film yourself walking barefoot for ten steps towards the camera and then ten steps away. Look for asymmetry. One foot turning out more than the other, reduced arm swing on one side, the head drifting, or an uneven sound pattern can all indicate where load is biased.

Common gait issues include:
- Heel whip, where the foot swings in or out after toe off, often linked to hip or knee control.
- Toe drag, which may show weakness or a coordination problem.
- Crossover gait, where the feet land on a narrow track, often tied to hip instability.
- A wide stance pattern, which can reflect balance concerns or core weakness.

Practical drills can help reset patterns:
- Walk barefoot on different textures to improve foot awareness.
- Use a metronome and adjust your pace to challenge timing.
- Practice clear toe off by pushing through the big toe.
- Walk upstairs slowly to encourage hip drive and walk downstairs with soft landings.
- Walk backwards gently to reveal hidden imbalances and reset patterns.

Mental cues also improve gait. Thinking about lengthening your stride slightly, allowing natural arm swing, or lifting the chest can improve mechanics in seconds.

A Real-life example

Steve is 49 and has a desk job. A former runner he now regularly keeps fit at his local gym. He came in with lower back pain and a history of recurring hamstring strains. When we analysed his gait, the issue became clear; he had minimal hip extension. His stride was short; his pelvis tilted forwards. He was lifting with his lower back, not pushing with his glutes. Basically, his glutes had taken early retirement, and nobody had told his spine.

A locked ankle from an old football injury had shortened his stride on one side, and the compensation caused asymmetrical pelvic loading. That one small ankle issue had been quietly sabotaging him for years.

Steve now jokes that he never thought fixing his back would start at his ankle. Welcome to physics, Steve.

Regen tips:

A wobble cushion or board gently trains the ankle to respond with more accuracy. It improves balance and restores the nervous system feedback that keeps your gait steady and your joints working in sequence while you go about everyday tasks such as brushing your teeth or taking a call.

Pillar 1 - Physics: The Structure of Healing

Terrain, Footwear and Daily Factors

Different surfaces can change gait. Softer ground demands greater balance and hard floors can increase impact forces. Your footwear plays a major role too as unsupportive shoes create asymmetry without you realising it. Over time, the body adapts to these changes so rotating your footwear and walking on varied terrain helps keep your system adaptable.

Fatigue also changes gait in ways that reveal underlying weaknesses. Early in the day you may walk smoothly but as tiredness sets in your natural patterns shift. Your stride length often reduces, foot placement becomes less precise, you might walk more heavily or drag your feet, and your hips may begin to drift or drop. These changes show where your body is struggling to manage load consistently.

Footwear offers useful clues as well. The wear pattern on your shoes shows how you distribute pressure with every step. Extra wear on one side of the heel suggests you land more heavily on that edge. Flattened forefoot wear can indicate limited toe off or reduced push through the big toe.

Fatigue and shoe wear patterns are early clues that your body is working harder in some areas than others and the next step is to use that information to guide how you move and what you prioritise.

If your stride shortens or becomes uneven when you are tired, it usually means a joint or muscle group is losing control under load. The immediate step is to slow your pace, pay attention to how you place each foot and give the body a chance to recover.

Patterns that only appear when you are tired are often the ones that lead to injury, so noticing them early helps you adjust before problems build.

When shoe wear indicates a problem, the practical response is to test the basics: can your ankle move freely, do your hips feel stiff, is one side working harder than the other? These simple checks help you understand where the imbalance might be starting.

If these patterns persist, the next logical step is a structured assessment. That could be a movement review, a gait analysis, or a professional evaluation that looks at how your joints, muscles and nervous system are coordinating. A trained eye can link those small clues to the underlying cause and show you how to correct them.

Gait as Emotional Feedback

Emotions influence gait. Research shows that slumped posture and short, shuffling steps reinforce low mood. Upright posture, steady rhythm and natural arm swing support a stronger emotional state. Movement affects mindset more than people realise.

Try it. Stand up straight with your chin up and chest open, see how that makes you feel and then slump over. You'll immediately notice the difference not only in how you feel but how your body moves.

Simple Physics: Torque, Angles and Joint Stress

The human body follows the same physical principles as every other structure in the world and those principles shape how your joints absorb force, how your muscles coordinate movement and how your tissues cope with daily life. Physics influences every step you take and every position you hold, which explains why some movements feel smooth while others feel heavy. When you understand how torque, angles and accumulated stress behave inside the body, you gain the ability to move with control rather than leaving your mechanics to habit and chance.

What Torque Means for the Body

Torque is rotational force and it appears whenever a joint turns. You experience it while turning your head, rotating through your spine, or pivoting through your feet during daily tasks. Torque itself is essential for movement. Problems arise when rotational force arrives from angles that place excessive strain on tissues that cannot accommodate that demand. For example, the knee is built to bend and straighten with only limited rotation, so turning the upper body while the foot stays

fixed creates force that the knee must absorb. Over time this strains ligaments and irritates cartilage. You've probably done these without even thinking:
- Twisting while lifting a shopping bag out of the car boot.
- Turning to speak to someone behind you without moving your feet.
- Playing with your kids on the floor and pivoting through the knee.

A practical correction is to let your feet turn with your body as you rotate so the movement travels from the ground upwards and the joints share the load in a more balanced way.

Angles Dictate Load

Every joint works best within a certain angle where movement feels smooth and load travels cleanly through the structure. When you move outside that angle repeatedly, leverage increases and the joint absorbs more force with every repetition. This shows up in everyday patterns that become so familiar you hardly notice them.

Common examples include:
- Knees drifting inwards during lower body movements, which increases stress on the inner knee.
- Shoulders rounding as the hours pass at a desk, which tightens the upper back and alters breathing.
- A head that gradually drifts forwards during concentration, which increases strain through the neck.

These positions shift weight into areas that cope poorly with sustained load, and the effect accumulates quietly over time

Pillar 1 - Physics: The Structure of Healing

The Power of Alignment

When your body sits in good alignment, force travels through you in a way that feels steady and predictable. The big muscles and joints take the workload they were built for and the more delicate areas stay settled, which makes everyday movement far more comfortable.

Helpful reference points include:
- Sitting with roughly a right angle at the hips, knees and elbows, which gives the spine a stable base and reduces unnecessary tension.
- Standing with the ears above the shoulders and the shoulders above the hips and ankles, which encourages the spine to behave like a supportive column.
- Lifting with a stable spine and active hips so the stronger muscles guide the movement and the lower back stays supported.

Small changes like these reduce strain before it accumulates and create healthier long-term mechanics.

The Modern Issue: Phone Neck

Screen use encourages the head to drift forwards, which greatly increases the load on the neck. The head weighs several kilograms and the further it travels from its neutral position, the heavier it becomes in mechanical terms. This changes how the entire upper body behaves. The muscles at the front of the neck shorten, the muscles at the back overwork and the upper back loses its natural efficiency. Over time this affects breathing, shoulder mobility and even balance, not to mention causing chronic neck ache and a potential hump as you get older.

A simple way to ease the pressure through the neck is to reset your head position. Sit or stand comfortably with the chest relaxed, then glide the head backwards without tipping it up or down. Hold the position for a few seconds and let the neck settle before releasing. Repeating this through the day, especially after long periods with screens, helps the deeper neck muscles wake up and guides the head back over the spine so the load feels lighter.

A helpful habit is to bring the phone towards eye level rather than lowering the head towards the device. This small change reduces hours of unnecessary strain each week.

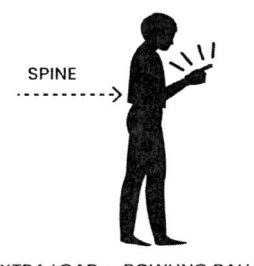

Joint Stress Builds in Many Forms

Heavy lifting rarely causes the only stress the body receives. Long periods of sitting with poor posture, repeated small movements during typing or texting, vibration through cycling or machinery and cumulative impact from hard surfaces all contribute to joint fatigue. These micro-stresses add up gradually and the body begins to compensate long before pain arrives.

Torque Chains and Force Leaks

The body moves as a connected system and each joint influences the next. When one area loses strength, freedom or stability, another area quietly absorbs more work. Stiff hips often push extra rotation into the lower back. A weakened or restricted ankle encourages the knees to take more load than they should. Limited movement around the shoulder blades changes how the neck and shoulders behave. These small shifts build patterns that shape how you move and how you feel over time.

You can feel this relationship through a simple standing twist. When the knees are free, the movement is smoother. When the knees are locked, everything becomes restricted because the force has nowhere to travel. The body experiences this every day when joints are limited by habit, posture or stiffness.

The spine works best when it remains stable and supported. When rotation or lifting comes from the spine rather than the hips and legs, the load centralises into a smaller area, which increases stress and reduces long-term resilience. Moving the feet during rotation, stacking the joints during daily tasks and allowing the larger muscles to support movement protects the entire chain.

Why following the principles of Physics matters

Physical rules shape how force travels, how joints age and how efficiently the body performs. These principles matter because regeneration relies on how well your body manages force over months and years. When movement follows cleaner angles and balanced pathways, tissues recover with less resistance, joints stay more agile and the nervous system works with a steadier baseline. Over time, these small mechanical changes protect your capacity to move with confidence, maintain strength and stay independent for longer.

This is the practical side of regeneration: it begins with how you stand, how you sit, how you lift and how you walk throughout the day. You are creating conditions that allow the body to keep renewing as opposed to wearing down.

MAI-Motion - Motion Analysis Intelligence

Regeneration isn't just about how you feel; it's about how you move, and the truth is, most of us have blind spots. You might think your posture is fine, or that you're walking evenly but the small compensations in your joints tell a different story. As I said at the beginning of the book, that's why I created *MAI-Motion - Motion Analysis Intelligence.*

To give you deeper insight and explain exactly how it works, MAI-Motion offers a comprehensive analysis of musculoskeletal movement, giving you a window into the dynamics of your joints, the patterns of your gait and the way your body absorbs and transfers force. Using 3D mesh technology, it captures your movement with unparalleled accuracy, creating a visual representation that shows exactly what's happening beneath the surface.

However, it doesn't stop there. MAI-Motion integrates with 3D volumetric MRI data, linking the way you move with the structural reality of your bones, muscles and connective tissue. That means we don't just see how your knee bends, we see how the cartilage, ligaments and muscle are influencing, or restricting, that motion.

On top of that, it's powered by artificial intelligence. Algorithms analyse the complex data, flagging asymmetries, weaknesses and risks, while also supporting treatment and rehabilitation strategies. It's decision support, not guesswork.

Why does this matter for regeneration – because it closes the loop. The pod provides the intervention, stimulation, acceleration and preservation. MAI-Motion provides the insight, the measurement, the feedback and the roadmap. One shows us what to do, the other proves what's working.

For you, it means precision.

For me, it means clarity.

For all of us, it means a tool that can assist in regeneration.

How We Use MAI-Motion

This is the part that genuinely excites me, because it represents a shift in how we can work with movement in real life. MAI-Motion exists because I wanted a clearer, more reliable way to understand how people actually move, not how they appear to move during a brief assessment.

MAI-Motion turns everyday movement into usable information. A short video, recorded on a smartphone, provides objective data on joint behaviour, timing, load transfer and movement consistency. This gives us a baseline we can return to, compare against and refine as the body adapts.

In practice, we use MAI-Motion as part of assessment, decision-making and follow-up. The analysis focuses on key movement markers: how joints travel through space, how well control is maintained, how force distributes across the body and how timing holds up under repetition or challenge. We also look at symmetry and centre of mass behaviour, because this is often where early breakdown appears long before pain becomes obvious.

What makes this powerful is not the technology itself but what it enables. MAI-Motion helps guide where to intervene, what to prioritise and when to progress. It allows us to test assumptions, confirm whether change is working and spot when compensation begins to creep back in under fatigue or load.

For the person being assessed, the impact is immediate. Seeing their own movement creates clarity and engagement. Progress becomes visible, measurable and motivating. Movement shifts from something that simply happens to something that can be shaped deliberately.

MAI-Motion supports regeneration by bringing consistency and feedback into the process. It helps us intervene earlier, track improvement with confidence and design movement strategies that hold up over time. This is where regeneration becomes practical, repeatable and personal.

You can feel this shift in awareness with a simple exercise. Film a side view of an unweighted squat and observe the knees, the hips, the spine and the point where control begins to drift. Watching yourself from the outside changes how the brain interprets movement. This creates a turning point. It is no longer about moving through habit, you begin to move with informed intention. This is the point where regeneration stops being a concept and starts becoming a process you can actively influence.

Download the software for free here:

Applying These Principles in Everyday Life

Understanding physics and movement patterns only matters if it changes what you do day to day. The real strain on your joints doesn't usually come from the gym or a single bad lift, it comes from how you carry shopping, sit at a desk, cook dinner or drive to work. These everyday movements are where small misalignments repeat often enough to shape long-term wear.

Before introducing tools that measure movement more precisely, it's important to recognise how these principles show up in ordinary life. Once you can see them there, everything that follows makes far more sense.

Real-Life Applications

Carrying Shopping or Children:

Mistake: Holding everything on one side. Hiking up the shoulder. Twisting the spine to balance the load.

Fix: Use both arms when possible. If carrying a child on one hip, alternate sides. Brace your core and avoid leaning away from the load.

Use backpacks rather than single-strap bags to distribute weight. If you must carry unevenly, counterbalance with opposite arm movement and walk with shorter steps to maintain stability.

Working at a Desk:

Mistake: Perching on the edge of the seat, slumping, or hunching over a laptop.

Fix: Have your feet flat, thighs parallel to the floor, arms relaxed at 90 degrees. Use a rolled towel for lumbar support. Raise the monitor to eye height. Take micro-breaks every 30 minutes to stand, stretch and reset. **Reminder**: If you're reading this hunched over, do a chin tuck now. Yes, now. Your future self will thank you.

If you're on video calls all day, stand for one, sit for the next, or walk while you talk.

Kitchen Tasks:

Mistake: Standing in one position while cooking or washing up, causing hip and back fatigue. If you've been stuck at the sink long enough to finish a podcast, change your stance.

Fix: Place one foot slightly in front of the other and switch every few minutes. Engage your glutes and keep your shoulders relaxed. If possible, rest one foot on a small block or drawer ledge to reduce lower back strain.

Driving:

Mistake: Slumping in the seat, reaching too far for the wheel, leaning on one armrest.

Fix: Bring the seat close enough to the pedals so your knees remain slightly bent. Support the lumbar spine. Place your hands on the wheel at positions 9 and 3 (on a clock face), elbows relaxed. Evenly distribute your weight across the hips.

If you drive long distances, shift positions every 30 minutes. Cruise control isn't laziness; it's lumbar therapy.

Household Chores:

Mistake: Twisting while vacuuming, mopping with one side, or bending from the back.

Fix: Use long, slow strokes, switch sides frequently and engage the whole body. Step into the movement instead of reaching. When picking things up, use a squat or lunge pattern. Get close to the item before lifting. Not only will this improve your joints, but you'll also get a bit more of a cardiac workout while doing so! Remember, good form isn't just for the gym.

How to Reduce Stress on Your Joints

Use stacked alignment: When standing or lifting, keep joints in line. Ear over shoulder, shoulder over hip, hip over knee,

knee over ankle. Think of your skeleton like a Jenga tower – if the blocks stack, it stands strong. If not, gravity wins.

Respect load and angle: Don't lift or twist from awkward positions. Physics doesn't care about your excuses. Twist under load and your joints will tell you about it.

Prioritise control over range: Being able to move further doesn't mean you should. Move where you can maintain control.

Build joint awareness drills:
Wrist circles (10 in each direction, daily)
Shoulder blade slides up and down the back
Ankle rolls while brushing your teeth (bonus: minty-fresh proprioception)

Vary your inputs: Change position every 20 minutes, alternating between sitting and standing. Wear different shoes and walk on a variety of surfaces.

Micro-Drills to Reprogramme Mechanics

- **Wall Angels**: Great for shoulder alignment.
    - Stand with your back flat to the wall, arms horizontal to your body.
    - Slide arms up and down while keeping contact.
- **Chair Squats**: These retrain one of the most fundamental human movements: sitting down and standing up. Done well, chair squats reinforce hip-driven movement, knee alignment and core control – all crucial for protecting joints and building functional strength.

- Practise sitting and standing without using hands. Keep your knees over your feet.

- **Counter Push-ups**: Builds core control and alignment for daily leaning motions. Builds upper body control and strengthens the core for daily tasks like leaning, reaching and pushing.
  - Stand facing your kitchen counter or a sturdy table.
  - Place hands shoulder-width apart on the edge. Step feet back until your body forms a straight line from head to heels.
  - Engage your core.
  - Lower your chest toward the counter, elbows tracking back.
  - Push back up to the start.
  - Do 10 slow, controlled reps.
  - Tip: Don't let your hips sag. Keep your neck long, not craning up or dropping down.

- **Glute Bridges**: Reset hip alignment and counteract long sitting periods.
  - Lie on your back, knees bent, feet flat and hip-width apart.
  - Arms by your sides.
  - Press into your heels, squeeze your glutes and lift your hips until your body forms a straight line from shoulders to knees.
  - Hold for 2–3 seconds at the top. Lower slowly.
  - Do 12–15 reps.
  - **Tip**: Avoid arching the lower back – the lift should come from your hips, not your spine.

- **Toe Taps While Seated**: These help to activate anterior tibialis and improve ankle control.
    - Sit upright on a chair, feet flat.
    - Keeping heels on the floor, lift your toes off the ground as high as you can.
    - Lower with control.
    - Repeat for 20 taps per foot.
    - **Tip**: If you can scroll Instagram, you can do toe taps. Multitask your way to better mechanics.

Tuning Into Internal Signals

Your body rarely shouts when something is wrong. It begins with gentle cues, almost like a polite cough from a butler trying to be helpful. A tight neck, a small twinge, a shift in how you stand. The sooner you notice these early messages, the less strain you place on your joints, tissues and nervous system.

Most people take action only when pain appears, however, pain is the final warning, not the first. Your body works like a dashboard: tension, temperature changes, altered breathing and disrupted rhythm are all early indicators. When they're ignored or suppressed, strain builds quietly until discomfort becomes unavoidable.

Why Listening Early Supports Regeneration

Pain is a delayed signal. Awareness is an early intervention.

Those subtle cues are the body's way of adjusting before more substantial stress accumulates. Regeneration depends on working with those early signs rather than overriding them. When you spot them early, you prevent the micro-wear that usually builds into long-term problems.

Imagine you're wearing new shoes for the day. The soreness you feel the next morning didn't appear overnight. You likely felt a small pinch by lunchtime, a shift in how you placed your weight, or even tension up through your ankle and calf. Those were your warning lights. Responding early reduces the load your body has to repair later. Carrying a comfortable spare pair or removing the shoes when you can is preventative mechanics.

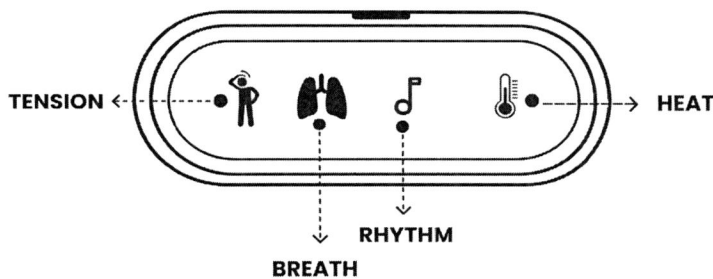

How Painkillers Mask Signals

Painkillers have their place, especially during acute episodes, however using them to "push through" discomfort hides vital information. When sensation is dulled, the body continues to move with the same underlying imbalance but with none of the feedback that would normally slow you down.

The cost is simple: you move more but you heal less.

Masked signals delay regeneration because the body cannot adapt around a problem it can no longer feel.

Real-Life Example

Lee experienced a spinal injury in her twenties that developed into long-term chronic pain. Over the years it expanded into further complications, including osteoarthritis. She worked long hours at a desk and relied heavily on painkillers to get through the day. What she didn't realise at the time was that her body was dealing with two problems at once: the physical strain of holding fixed positions for hours and a nervous system that had learned to expect pain so it could receive the chemical reward of medication.

When additional health issues pushed her pain to a severe level, she eventually had to come off the painkillers, a process that was far from easy. After several months, something unexpected happened. Her pain reduced and her movement improved because she could finally hear her body's natural signals again, rather than the artificial feedback loop created by long-term medication.

Important note: Always speak to a qualified professional before stopping any medication. Even over-the-counter pain relief needs guidance if you've been taking it regularly for a long time.

What Internal Signals Actually Look Like

Tension

Tension is more than stress; it's an early sign of overwork. It gathers in the neck, jaw, shoulders, lower back or hips when the body tries to stabilise without the support it needs.

Try this: lift your shoulders towards your ears and then let them drop. That difference is your reset point.

Breath

Your breath reveals your nervous system immediately. Shallow chest breathing suggests strain; calm diaphragmatic breathing signals safety.

If you cannot hold a conversation while doing so, your system is carrying unnecessary load.

Red Flags Worth Paying Attention To

- Always shifting onto the same leg
- Jaw clenching during concentration
- Holding breath while lifting, reaching or standing
- Always carrying a phone or bag on the same side
- Bracing when sitting or standing instead of using steady strength

Repeated throughout the week, these patterns create long-term imbalance. There is no judgement here; it simply means your body is due some attention.

The Sensory Systems Guiding You

Your brain relies on three inputs that shape movement:
- **Proprioception**: knowing where your joints are without looking
- **Vestibular input**: balance, orientation and stability
- **Visual cues:** your posture shifts to match where your eyes go

Any disruption to one system – tiredness, lighting, stress – changes your movement pattern.

Home Tests to Build Awareness

1. One-Leg Balance Test
Stand barefoot on one leg with eyes closed. Hold for 10 seconds. Repeat on both sides. If one side feels very different, your balance and proprioception need support.

2. Breath and Movement Drill
Walk slowly while breathing only through your nose. Add natural arm swings. Any increase in tension or breathlessness highlights nervous system strain.

3. Tension Scan
Before bed, lie flat and mentally scan from head to toe. Release tension when possible. Make a very short note of anything that repeats: "Jaw tight again today."

Daily Practices to Tune In

1. Micro-Journaling (one minute)
Note where you felt tight, where you held breath and what movements felt off.

2. Movement Check-Ins (11am & 3pm)
Three breaths, shoulder rolls, gentle twists, relaxed jaw. These small resets prevent cumulative strain.

3. End-of-Day Reset
Feet elevated for five minutes while breathing slowly. This encourages passive recovery and helps the nervous system settle.

The Female Physiology Note
- Hormonal changes affect joint laxity, stability and recovery.
- Ovulation increases elasticity, raising injury risk.
- Menstruation can lower energy and shift perception.
- Perimenopause and menopause reduce tissue repair speed.

Understanding these shifts allows you to adapt movement without self-blame.

This Is Practical Regeneration

Regeneration relies on small adjustments made early, long before problems become deeply embedded. When you pay attention to signals as they appear and act on them, the body maintains alignment more easily, reduces unnecessary strain and restores balance with far less effort.

It works the same way you would review a document before sending it. A tiny correction made early saves hours of repair later. The moment you notice tension, altered rhythm, breath changes, or a shift in how you move, you have an opportunity to guide your body back towards healthier patterns. Over time, those early responses create stronger mechanics, steadier movement and a foundation for long-term resilience that supports the quality of life you want to keep as you age.

Regen tips:

A simple desk timer acts as a cue to check in with your body before tension builds. When it goes off every ninety minutes, stand, breathe, roll your shoulders and let your system reset. These small interruptions help you stay aware of how you are sitting, breathing and holding yourself, and also they prevent the subtle shutdown that creeps in when you stay in one position for too long.

Energy Input and the Physical Signals You Might Be Missing

When we talk about energy in the context of regeneration and physics, we're not talking about feeling tired after lunch. We're talking about the real currency of movement: how force moves through you, how heat builds and how recovery works when the system plays fair. Every second of the day, your body is running an energy economy.

Energy input is the foundation of everything your body does: walking, healing, thinking, even standing still. Every cell in your body runs on energy. Every muscle contraction, every nerve signal, every repair process depends on energy being delivered, transferred and used correctly.

Here's the important bit: when energy flow is smooth, you feel light, strong and efficient. When it leaks, you feel heavy, tired and slower than a Monday morning.

Pillar 1 - Physics: The Structure of Healing

What Is Energy, Physically Speaking?

In physics, energy is the capacity to do work. In your body, that translates to the capacity to move, function and regenerate. There are several types of energy relevant here:

- **Kinetic energy**: The energy of movement – walking, bending, lifting.
- **Potential energy**: Stored energy in muscles, joints and tendons. Think of a spring just before it snaps back.
- **Thermal energy**: Heat generated by movement and friction – such as during exercise or inflammation.
- **Chemical energy**: Stored in food, converted by the body into ATP (adenosine triphosphate), the fuel your cells run on.
- **Electromagnetic energy**: Nerve impulses, brain function and muscle firing all involve electrical signals.

This is physics running beneath your skin. If energy isn't transferred efficiently your body works harder for less return. It means more friction, more fatigue and more wear.

Signs You're Losing Energy

Think of your energy system like a road. Smooth flow means effortless travel. Block it with bad posture or stiff joints and you'll have traffic jams and detours. That's when your body burns extra fuel just to keep moving.

Physical signals you might be missing energy:
- **Heaviness in limbs** during basic tasks like walking up stairs.

- **Delayed muscle activation** – muscles that should fire first lag behind.
- **Excess heat** in a specific joint or area – a sign of friction and inefficiency.
- **Unexplained fatigue** after minimal movement.
- **Audible joint noises** – creaks, cracks, or pops can suggest misdirected force.

These are not just quirks of ageing. They're red flags that your body isn't transferring energy effectively.

Energy Pathways in Motion

Energy needs clear, efficient routes to get from Point A to Point B.

Here's the important bit: when the route's blocked, energy doesn't stop, it finds a workaround and these cost more. More load creates more stress and more fuel burned for the same output.

Take walking, for example. The energy to propel you forwards should start at the foot, travel through the ankle, knee, hip, spine and shoulder. If your ankle is stiff or your hip doesn't extend properly, the system compensates. Other muscles take over and more energy is used for less return.

It's like running a Formula 1 engine on flat tyres. The power's there but you're dragging through every corner.

That's when regeneration slows down, because your energy is being spent just holding things together, not healing.

Improving Energy Efficiency

The goal isn't to generate more energy; your body already makes plenty. The real win is wasting less.

1. Tissue Quality
Scar tissue, adhesions and stiff fascia (connective tissue) block smooth energy transfer. Movement becomes jerky and inefficient.

Fix: Daily mobility work, foam rolling, massage, stretching after heat (shower or short walk) to increase elasticity.

2. Joint Stack and Alignment
If joints are stacked properly, energy travels through them efficiently. Misalignment creates torque and resistance.

Fix: Posture resets and core activation drills.

3. Muscle Firing Order
Muscles must activate in the right order, glutes before hamstrings and scapula before deltoid. When this order breaks, energy is lost to compensation.

Fix: Pre-activity priming. Try glute bridges before a walk, scapular wall slides before upper body workouts and so on. Think of it like cueing up the orchestra before the concert. You want the violins (glutes) in before the tambourines (hamstrings) crash in.

4. Breathing and Oxygenation
Poor breathing mechanics limit oxygen delivery which is a key part of energy creation.

Fix: Breathe through your nose. Use diaphragmatic breathing (belly rise). Slow your exhalations to engage parasympathetic recovery.

Real-Life example

Mark, 52, came in complaining of fatigue and recurring calf tightness. He exercised regularly and had no major injuries however, a gait analysis revealed his right hip wasn't extending fully. That meant every step required his calves and lower back to work overtime. Energy wasn't travelling up the chain so his muscles were doing work his joints should have handled.

We added hip extension drills, corrected his stance and taught him breathing resets to activate his core. Within two weeks, the calf pain had eased and his energy returned.

He didn't need more sleep, pain injections or surgery. He needed mechanics.

Your Own Energy Audit
Start tracking the small signals:
- Which movements feel sluggish?
- Which joints always feel hot or stiff?
- Do you feel more tired after sitting than standing?
- Where do you carry tension, neck, jaw, lower back?

Pillar 1 - Physics: The Structure of Healing

Use a simple log:

Time	Activity	Fatigue Level (1-10)	Notable Symptoms
9am	Walking dog	4	Left ankle tight
3pm	Zoom call	7	Neck ache, yawning

Patterns tell the story. You don't need a lab test for this, just attention and honesty.

Note - Don't Confuse Energy With Inflammation

Heat is a natural byproduct of energy use. Muscles warm up when they're working efficiently, that's normal, but a joint that feels hot to the touch, especially when at rest, could signal inflammation.

Energy heat is general, temporary and improves with movement (think of the warmth you feel after walking or stretching).

Rule of thumb: if the heat lingers long after you've stopped moving, it's a warning sign.

Inflammation heat is localised, persistent and often paired with swelling, stiffness, or pain. It usually gets worse after rest, not better.

If your knee feels warm after a hike and settles with gentle movement or elevation, it's likely energy-related but if that same heat lingers for hours and worsens overnight, you're looking at a possible inflammatory response.

Rule of thumb: If heat comes with pain, swelling, or stiffness, investigate. If it comes with movement and eases with recovery, it's likely a good sign your tissues are active and engaged.

Micro-Habits to Boost Input and Efficiency

- **Breath ladders**: Inhale for 3 steps, exhale for 3 steps during walking.
- **Reset drills:** Every 2 hours: shoulder rolls, hip circles, standing glute squeeze.
- **Contrast therapy**: Finish your shower with 30 seconds cold; this helps to wake up your circulation.
- **Barefoot balance**: Train your feet. Spend 5 minutes barefoot on grass or carpet. Try toe spreading, towel scrunches with your toes and single-leg standing. The stronger your feet, the better your energy transfer.
- **Active rest**: Lying on the floor with legs elevated for 5 mins boosts recovery.

Regeneration Isn't Speed-Cooking

The Physics Lesson Nobody Wants to Hear (But Needs to)

You wouldn't throw a roast in the oven at 400°C for an hour and expect a Michelin star, you'd expect inedible offerings. Yet, that's how many people treat their bodies. Hammer it with intensity, zero patience and wonder why it fails.

Here's the deal:
- **Load + Time = Adaptation.**
- Get the ratio wrong and you either burn out (overload) or stay raw (underload).

Pillar 1 - Physics: The Structure of Healing

Think of it like this:
- **2 hours of HIT (High Intensity Training)?** That's max effort every session, no recovery. You'll get results, sure. But they'll be injuries, inflammation and exhaustion.
- **4 x 30-minute sessions?** Controlled load, sustained over time. That's where regeneration happens – steady and efficient.

Physics says energy transfer isn't instant. Your tissues adapt gradually. Push too hard and the energy doesn't build structure, it destroys it.

Recipe for Regeneration
- **Start low, build slow.** You don't hit max load on day one.
- **Measure the inputs.** Load, frequency, recovery. Get them wrong and you're serving burnt offerings.
- **Patience = Power.** Controlled stress signals repair. Chaos signals breakdown.

So next time you think "more is better", picture that lump of blackened chicken.

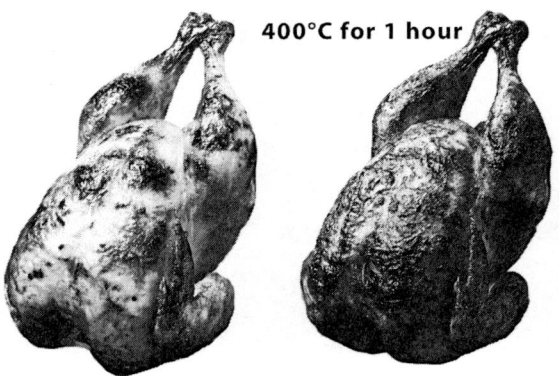

400°C for 1 hour

180°C for 1.45 hours

Final Thought

Energy is your hidden currency. You trade it for every movement, every breath, every repair your body makes.

If you feel worn out, it's not just about working harder, it's about working smarter. Efficient mechanics, smart breathing, joint alignment and daily resets all improve your energy economy.

What Is Grounding (and Why Should You Care)?

Grounding, or earthing, as it's often called, is the practice of reconnecting your body to the earth's natural electrical field. The concept is simple: physical contact with the ground helps neutralise excess positive charge in your body.

Ancient humans didn't need this conversation as they walked barefoot, slept on natural surfaces, touched soil every day. Now, we live in concrete jungles, wear rubber-soled shoes and spend 90% of our time indoors. We're constantly surrounded by Wi-Fi, EMFs (Electro Magnetic Fields) and artificial environments but we almost never touch the earth.

Wellness influencers turned grounding into an aesthetic: think barefoot yoga on the beach, but beyond this there's real science behind why it matters.

Practical Ways to Ground Yourself

The question most people ask is how to begin grounding without escaping to the countryside. The answer is far simpler than it appears. Your body responds the moment it receives direct contact with natural surfaces, and those opportunities exist in ordinary, everyday environments.

- **Barefoot walking:** Grass, soil or sand work well for grounding because the contact is immediate and uninterrupted. Twenty to thirty minutes creates a strong effect, although even a few minutes makes a noticeable difference once it becomes part of your routine.
- **Natural contact:** Gardening without gloves, sitting on the grass or lying on the beach all create the same response. The benefit comes from the connection rather than the scenery, which means small, regular moments matter.
- **Water grounding:** Swimming in natural water allows the skin to conduct the earth's electrical potential quickly and consistently, making it one of the most effective forms of grounding.

Winter weather, city living or long working hours can create limitations, yet the principle remains the same. Conductive materials provide a pathway for charge to disperse so the body can settle. A grounding mat under the feet during work creates a route for steady discharge. Conductive bedding, woven with fibres such as silver or carbon, allows the body to connect to the earth throughout the night, which is often when electrical balance plays a crucial role in deep recovery. Grounding socks, straps, or adhesive patches support the same process and can be especially helpful during travel or injury rehabilitation when irritation or inflammation needs to be managed carefully.

A sunrise walk or sunset on the beach provides the most natural experience and remains my personal preference. However, many people live and work in environments where that is not realistic and this is where technology offers a useful bridge rather than a compromise.

Grounding is not an exercise in perfection; it is a practical way to restore balance in a system that spends most of its time under electrical strain. Even modest amounts of contact can shift how the body feels for the rest of the day.

Grounding and Recovery: Why Athletes Swear by It

Elite athletes and performance labs have been experimenting with grounding for years because it works. Post-training grounding has been linked to reduced muscle soreness, faster recovery and better sleep quality. When your nervous system calms down and inflammation drops, your body can repair instead of staying stuck in fight-or-flight mode.

Combine that with smart chemistry, hydration, protein, omega-3s and you've got a recovery stack that beats any expensive "detox" fad.

Think about the last time you were in nature – that sudden deep breath you let out, the feeling of tension leaving you – that's grounding.

How Does This Fit Into My Approach?

We live in a world that never powers down. Screens, signals, artificial light – your body is bombarded by input every waking hour. Grounding is one of the simplest ways to unplug your system without moving to the mountains. Do it consistently and you'll feel the difference, not in months but in days.

It costs nothing, it requires no supplements and the side effects are lower stress, better sleep, less pain. That's a prescription I'll write all day long.

You might be wondering, "If I start grounding, do I still need all the other strategies?" Here's the honest answer: grounding isn't a silver bullet. When you combine electrical balance with chemistry and physics however, you create synergy that moves you closer to the goal: youthful function, resilience and longevity.

Why It Matters for Longevity

Here's the big picture: inflammation and oxidative stress accelerate ageing, but anything that reduces that load slows the clock. You can throw pills at the problem but if your electrical system is out of balance, you're patching cracks in the foundation. Grounding fixes the base.

Remember this: longevity isn't just chemistry or physics; it's the combination of both. Grounding is where those two worlds meet.

So tomorrow morning, take your coffee outside. Stand barefoot on the grass and feel silly if you want but that small act is a hard reset for your biology and a step towards a future of health.

You now know that staying young isn't just about what you put in your body. It's also about how you connect it to the world beneath your feet.

The effects of heat waves, sound waves and electromagnetic fields on the body

Energy interacts with the body in several different forms, each type influencing how tissues behave, recover and adapt. Heat waves change temperature within muscles and joints, shifting circulation, flexibility and the rate at which cells carry out their work, while sound waves travel through the body as gentle vibrations that encourage fluid movement, pressure changes and a gradual easing of tension. Electromagnetic fields shape the way electrical signals travel through nerves, influence cellular charge and support the balance that allows tissues to coordinate movement and repair. These forms of energy follow clear physical rules and once those rules are understood, they become practical tools that can support recovery in predictable ways.

Heat, sound and electromagnetic fields influence the way energy moves within tissues, guiding circulation, nerve activity and cellular responsiveness. When these energies are delivered with structure and purpose, they create conditions that support repair, enhance comfort and help the body organise itself more effectively during activity.

A simple starting point is the cell itself. Mitochondria, which are the body's microscopic power stations, convert oxygen and nutrients into usable energy and their performance depends on temperature, oxygen delivery, electrical charge and the mechanical environment around them. Heat, sound and electromagnetic waves all influence these factors at the same time, with heat increasing mitochondrial activity, sound waves supporting fluid movement around tissues and electromagnetic fields shaping the electrical gradients that cells rely on to produce energy consistently.

Early signs of uneven energy flow often appear in the way a person moves or feels through the day. It's worth you noticing whether one side absorbs load differently during a stride, whether the body braces or shifts weight without conscious awareness, whether the same shoulder or hip stiffens regularly, or whether mornings begin with rigidity that only settles as movement and warmth increase. Each pattern reflects a different imbalance in temperature, fluid movement, electrical signalling or load distribution.

Energy-based therapies offer practical ways to influence these patterns. Heat waves support circulation, elasticity and the warm, responsive state tissues need for healthy movement. Sound waves assist fluid flow, pressure changes and the gentle release of tension in deeper layers. Electromagnetic fields guide nerve communication, stabilise electrical gradients and help cells maintain the steady internal state required for repair and coordination. Each of these inputs contributes to the body's natural ability to reorganise and restore itself, provided they are matched thoughtfully to the situation at hand.

Selecting the right form of energy for each issue is an essential part of using these tools well. Heat supports areas that benefit from improved circulation and flexibility, sound waves support tissues that require fluid movement or gentle decompression and electromagnetic fields support regions where nerve activity or cellular stability needs guidance. When these choices are made with clarity, they create an environment in which the body can respond with greater consistency, efficiency and resilience.

Energy interacts with biology through physical principles that are reliable and predictable and understanding these principles allows each wave, field and frequency to become part of a regenerative environment that supports comfort, movement and long-term health.

How Therapies Connect to Physics

These therapies work through the same physical forces that shape movement and recovery: light, heat, vibration, electrical charge and electromagnetic fields. Each one interacts with tissue in a measurable way and when wavelength, temperature, frequency, or field strength are applied with the right timing, the body responds by improving circulation, increasing cellular energy production, supporting the nervous system and guiding tissue repair. They follow the same principles of energy flow introduced earlier and provide structured, practical methods that help the body recover more efficiently while building long-term resilience.

They sit here in the physics chapter because each uses a physical input that the body understands. These forces shape how energy moves, how cells behave and how tissues repair. When applied with intention, they improve circulation, guide cellular activity and support the mechanics of repair. They translate physics into practical tools that help the body regenerate more effectively.

Red Light Therapy

Red light therapy uses specific wavelengths, most commonly around 660 and 850 nanometres, that travel beneath the skin and influence how mitochondria produce ATP (adenosine triphosphate). Mitochondria act as the body's internal power stations and ATP fuels every process that keeps tissue healthy, responsive and capable of repair. When red light reaches these power stations, it supports a steadier and more efficient release of energy, which creates the foundations for improved recovery. The research across wound healing, joint comfort, sports recovery, inflammation and skin quality is extensive and the benefits tend to build with regular exposure because mitochondria respond best to consistent stimulation.

Heat and Cold

Heat affects the body by increasing circulation, encouraging soft tissues to relax and improving the movement of fluid around joints. Warmth alters the viscosity of the fluids that support movement, allowing muscles and connective tissue to become more flexible and responsive. Infrared heat works even deeper, reaching layers that benefit from increased oxygen delivery and metabolic activity. Cold has a complementary role by guiding fluid movement away from irritated areas, calming swelling and settling tissues after physical stress. Cryotherapy (the use of extremely low temperatures) provides a rapid temperature shift that influences both circulation and the nervous system, often leaving people with a sense of clarity and restored energy. The value of heat and cold lies in the control they provide, allowing each region of the body to receive the specific temperature environment it needs at that moment in the recovery process.

Laser Therapy

Laser therapy delivers highly focused light at greater intensity than red light, enabling deeper penetration and more targeted influence on tissue. It is often used for tendons, ligaments and joints, where precise stimulation supports mobility and reduces long-standing discomfort. Laser therapy encourages cells to re-engage with the repair process, which is particularly helpful in conditions that have developed slowly or where tissue has reached a plateau. Clinical evidence shows consistent improvements in pain, mobility and functional outcomes, making this a valuable tool for structured recovery plans.

Shockwave Therapy

Shockwave therapy uses high-energy sound waves that pass through tissue and create deep mechanical pressure changes. These waves influence dense or slow-healing structures by increasing circulation, stimulating cellular activity and breaking down areas of stiffness or calcification. Sound waves reach tissue layers that are often difficult to influence through manual therapy alone and they provide a strong stimulus that encourages regeneration where progress has stalled. This is why shockwave therapy is frequently used for tendon issues, plantar fasciitis, calcific shoulder problems and other conditions that require direct activation. The intensity of the sensation reflects the depth at which the waves travel and the clinical outcomes show consistent, measurable benefits, especially in cases where long-standing discomfort has limited movement or performance.

Sound Therapy

Low-frequency sound therapy uses vibration to influence the flow of fluid, the behaviour of connective tissue and the tone of muscles. These vibrations travel easily through the body's water-rich tissues, supporting gradual releases of tension and encouraging a shift toward a calmer nervous system state. Alongside clinical approaches, there are also sound baths and gong-based sessions where practitioners use sustained, repeating frequencies to guide the body into deeper relaxation. These sound waves influence breathing, muscle guarding and emotional tension, making them helpful when a person is recovering from physical stress, high-intensity training, or periods of cognitive overload. The shared principle across all forms of sound therapy is that vibration provides a stable pattern the body can follow, which supports clarity, recovery and nervous system regulation.

PEMF (Pulsed Electromagnetic Fields)

PEMF therapy applies magnetic pulses that interact with cells at an electrical level. These pulses influence ion channels, cellular signalling, circulation and the balance of electrical charge that supports tissue coordination. Hospitals have used PEMF for many years to support bone recovery and advances in the technology now allow similar principles to be applied to soft tissue and joint health. The improvements tend to build gradually, making PEMF particularly valuable for long-term support after injury, surgery, or prolonged periods of strain.

It enhances the internal environment of tissues by improving communication between cells and supporting the steady release of energy.

Terahertz (THz)

Terahertz occupies the space between infrared and microwave on the electromagnetic spectrum and interacts strongly with water molecules. Since water governs nutrient transport, oxygen delivery, waste removal and cellular communication, terahertz represents an emerging field with significant regenerative potential. Early studies suggest that terahertz waves may influence fluid organisation, circulation and tissue oxygenation in subtle but meaningful ways. Research teams are also exploring possible roles in inflammation control, early disease detection and cellular behaviour. As understanding grows, terahertz is likely to become an increasingly important part of regenerative science.

Electrical Muscle Stimulation (EMS)

Electrical Muscle Stimulation delivers controlled electrical impulses that create muscle contractions, supporting circulation, strength and joint stability without placing additional mechanical load on the body. These impulses mirror natural nerve signals, allowing muscles to stay active during recovery or periods of limited movement, which helps preserve healthy movement patterns and prevents compensation. EMS is sometimes thought to be similar to TENS, although the two technologies serve different purposes. TENS guides sensory nerves in a way that influences how discomfort is processed, whereas EMS focuses on producing rhythmic muscle contractions that support repair, coordination and long-term function. EMS becomes even more effective when tissues are already warm, well-oxygenated and electrically balanced, making it an important companion to other energy therapies.

How These Therapies Are Delivered

All of these therapies are provided by trained specialists who understand the timing, intensity and clinical reasoning behind their use. Physiotherapists, medical laser practitioners, osteopaths, sports rehabilitators, regenerative clinicians and sound therapy practitioners guide the process to ensure each therapy is matched to the individual, their condition and their stage of recovery. This allows the energy being delivered to work with the body's natural rhythms, ensuring comfort, clarity and effective repair.

What Should You Actually Do With This?

Each energy therapy plays a different role in recovery. When you understand what each one supports, you can match the right method to your needs instead of guessing. Think of this as a set of tools that help your body respond more efficiently.
- Red light supports recovery after training or surgery because it encourages mitochondria to release energy more efficiently, which strengthens tissue repair.
- Heat eases morning stiffness by improving circulation, while controlled cold settles inflammation later in the day when swelling becomes more active.
- Shockwave therapy suits long-standing tendon problems such as plantar fasciitis, Achilles tendinopathy, or tennis elbow because it delivers a focused mechanical stimulus that encourages slow-healing fibres to reorganise.

- Laser therapy helps when joints feel irritated or inflamed, particularly knees, shoulders and fingers, because it delivers concentrated light deeper into tissue to support cellular activity.
- Sound or vibration is valuable after stress or exercise because it influences fluid movement and guides the nervous system toward a calmer, more regulated state.
- PEMF provides steady support for joint discomfort since magnetic fields help maintain the electrical behaviour cells rely on to repair.
- Terahertz sits at the edge of emerging research and is worth watching as new evidence continues to grow.
- EMS supports muscle health during recovery by keeping fibres active, maintaining circulation and protecting movement patterns when exercise is limited.

When these therapies are used thoughtfully, they support the body's natural cycles of repair. They do not replace movement; they reinforce it. The real advantage appears when you understand what your body is telling you through posture, load, rhythm and ease of motion and then choose the energy input that complements those signals.

Introducing The Regen PhD Pod

After years of watching patients move between treatments that worked well in isolation but failed to function as a coherent system, I wanted to design an environment rather than another tool, one in which energy, heat, light, magnetics and gentle mechanical input are coordinated as part of a single, organised approach. By bringing these elements together in a controlled setting, timing can be managed deliberately and recovery supported in a way that does not depend on will-power, sustained effort or perfect compliance.

The therapies listed above each provide a specific benefit when used alone. However, as you're already starting to see, the body doesn't operate in isolated compartments. It responds best when energy, heat, light, magnetics and mechanical input are coordinated rather than scattered.

This is the concept that shaped the Regen PhD Pod. Instead of adding one energy at a time and hoping they work together, the Pod brings these principles into a single controlled environment where timing, intensity and layering can be managed precisely.

Here is how the Pod reflects the same mechanisms as the individual therapies from a physics perspective:

Each energy works in its own way when used on its own, yet the body responds best when these forms of energy support each other. This is what shaped the design of the Pod. Instead of adding heat one day, light the next and vibration when you remember, the Pod brings these elements together in a single environment where the timing, intensity and interaction are carefully controlled.

The principles behind red light appear in the *Cell Light Photon System*, which delivers specific wavelengths that encourage mitochondria to produce energy more efficiently. This creates the same benefits as clinical red light therapy but through a broader and more evenly distributed field.

The benefits of heat therapy are reflected in the *Bio-Carbon Resonance and Regen-FIR systems*, where steady, consistent warmth reaches deep into tissue and supports circulation, relaxation and recovery across the entire body rather than concentrating on one small area. Think of it like switching on a slow, even heat across the whole body so tissue unwinds, blood moves and recovery becomes easier without needing to rotate a heat pack from place to place.

The effect of sound and vibration is echoed in the *Bio-Harmonic Vibration platform*, which creates gentle rhythmic motion throughout the body and helps fluid shift more freely, supporting relaxation and nervous system balance in a way that mirrors advanced sound-based therapies.

Pillar 1 - Physics: The Structure of Healing

Magnetic field principles are carried through the rotating *PEMF system*, which guides the body's natural electrical behaviour and encourages tissues to repair in a more organised and efficient way, rather than focusing magnetic pulses on a single point.

Emerging ideas from terahertz research are brought into the *THz Quantum Wave* component, which interacts with water within the body and may support cellular communication and tissue hydration in ways early studies are beginning to highlight. People often notice that joints move more smoothly and areas that normally feel "puffy" or irritated settle more quickly.

The goals behind EMS are represented in the *Active Recovery Elements*, which encourage light micro-activation, preserve healthy muscle patterns and support circulation without requiring full muscular effort, making it especially helpful when someone is recovering or unable to exercise fully.

When these components work together, they create a physical environment that helps the body relax, recover, reorganise and regain balance. The intention is simple: to give your body the right signals at the right time so that regeneration becomes easier and more predictable. Each element inside the Pod mirrors the logic of the individual therapies but allows them to interact, layer and support each other at the same time. Instead of deciding between heat, light, magnetics, movement, or vibration, the Pod provides them together in a sequence that respects the body's own physics.

The result is a setting where tissues receive multiple aligned inputs simultaneously, which can help the body settle, recover and reorganise more efficiently than when these therapies are used one at a time.

When I designed this, my goal was simple: to create a system that feels like giving your cells a first-class upgrade while you just lie there thinking, "Wow, this is magic". Except it's not; it's science.

Key Wellness Benefits:

- Relieves muscle and joint tension
- Improves sleep quality
- Boosts energy levels and mental clarity
- Promotes physical recovery
- Encourages nervous system balance

Why stop at a spa day when your body can have a physics upgrade?

Part of a Bigger System

The Pod doesn't stand alone. It's part of the wider Regen PhD ecosystem, integrated with diagnostic tools like MAI-Motion. It also includes bone scan and genetic testing, plus expert programmes (all to be discussed as we move through the book). It's my physical proof of the principle: regeneration by design and practical regeneration by building systems.

Chapter Summary

The chapter explored how physical forces shape everything your body does each day: how you move, how you hold yourself, how you absorb energy and how you recover. Once you understand these forces, you can guide your body towards better resilience with far more clarity and confidence.

You learned to see movement as information. Gait patterns, joint angles, sequencing, breath behaviour and balance all reveal how your system is managing load. MAI-Motion made this even clearer. By measuring torque pathways, timing, symmetry and how force travels through each joint in the chain, it transforms movement analysis from guesswork into meaningful data. Combined with the C.R.A.F.T. model, you now have a framework that shows where efficiency thrives and where it quietly breaks down.

Posture and gravity work better when you see them as something you manage rather than something that happens to you. The way your head, spine, hips, knees and feet organise themselves affects how load travels through your body and which structures take on the work.

Energy also became a living concept. Heat, light, vibration, electrical activity, magnetics and breath all influence how cells repair, how tissues communicate and how the nervous system settles. These forces are measurable, predictable and deeply relevant to how regeneration unfolds.

This is where the Regen PhD Pod fits. It combines the same physics explored in this chapter, bringing them together with precision and structure:

- **Light energy** supports mitochondrial efficiency
- **Thermal resonance** improves circulation and tissue ease
- **Vibration and rhythmic motion** encourage fluid movement
- **Electromagnetic fields** guide cellular repair
- **Terahertz waves** influence tissue hydration and communication

Light + Heat + Sound + Magnet + Vibration

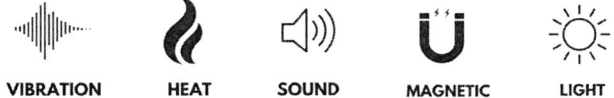

Each element mirrors the science behind heat, light, magnetics, movement and energy transfer. Instead of receiving these inputs one at a time, the Pod layers them in a controlled sequence so the body receives clear, coherent signals that support regeneration.

Across the chapter, one core theme emerged: the body responds to the forces it experiences. When those forces align well, movement becomes smoother, tension reduces, energy improves and

Pillar 1 - Physics: The Structure of Healing

recovery becomes easier. Small changes in rhythm, posture, sequencing and load distribution accumulate into meaningful long-term progress.

Regeneration grows from understanding how force moves through you, how your joints respond to load and how your rhythms guide movement. When you work with those principles instead of against them, the body restores more easily and the effort you put in actually pays off.

Practical Section

Movement Self-Checks (Quick & Telling)

You don't need a lab coat for these. Just honesty, a mirror and your phone camera.

1. Gait Footage Test
   - [ ] Film yourself walking towards and away from the camera, barefoot if you can. Notice:
   - [ ] Whether one foot lands heavier
   - [ ] If your shoulders move evenly
   - [ ] Whether your hips stay level or drift
   - [ ] If your head stays centred
   - [ ] Whether your arm swing looks natural or tense

2. Mirror Posture Scan
   - [ ] Stand barefoot and relaxed. Look for:
   - [ ] One shoulder sitting higher
   - [ ] A head tilt or forward head position
   - [ ] Hands turning inwards (tight shoulders)
   - [ ] Knees locked or soft

3. Toe Touch and Overhead Reach
　　☐ Can you touch your toes without bending your knees or bracing?
　　☐ Can you lift both arms overhead without your ribs flaring or your back arching?

4. Single-Leg Stability
　　☐ Stand barefoot on one leg for 30 seconds.
　　☐ Notice if you clench your jaw, wobble, or flare your arms out to balance.

Do these once a month. They're your personal MOT for movement and they tell you exactly where attention is needed before anything slips.

Don't walk into the consultant's office with "My back hurts" and hope for the best. Go in prepared and you'll get far better answers.

Try asking:
- "What's working harder than it should to support this area?"

　　_____

　　_____

- "Can you show me which parts are tight and which parts need more strength?"

　　_____

　　_____

- "Am I moving with rhythm or relying on tension?"

- "What's the first adjustment you'd make to improve my movement pattern?"

- "What steps help this stay settled over the long term?"

- "How smooth is my movement when you assess it?"

- "Have you measured it so we can track progress?"

These questions shift the conversation from symptoms to understanding. The right practitioner will welcome them because they open the door to better guid ance, clearer feedback and a plan that actually supports regeneration.

Daily Tools That Actually Help

You don't need to kit out a home gym. The right tools, used with intention, are enough.

Tool	What It Does	When to Use
Wobble Cushion or Board	Builds ankle control, balance, nervous system feedback	While brushing teeth or on calls
Standing Desk or Laptop Riser	Restores spine alignment, resets hip flexors	Alternate hourly – don't ditch your chair, just move more
Pilates Ball	Activates core and postural muscles, improves balance	Sit on it instead of a chair for short bursts (20 mins max), especially when typing or doing admin
Foam Roller / Massage Ball	Frees up stiff fascia that's disrupting flow	Use post-work or post-walk
Timer for Desk Breaks	Stops creeping shutdown	90 mins: stand, breathe, shoulder roll, march

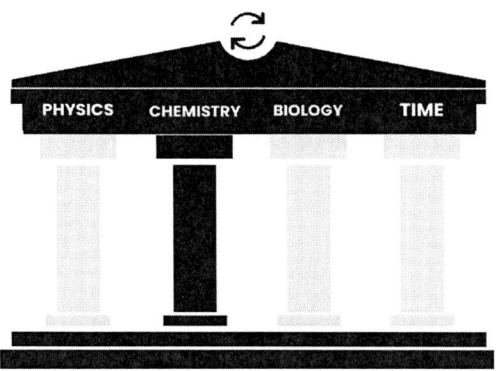

Pillar 2 - Chemistry: The Invisible War

"What you put in, what you break down, what you excrete – it all speaks."

The art of healing comes from nature, not from the physician. Therefore, the physician must start from nature, with an open mind.

Paracelsus

Medicine is chemistry in action

You can't see chemistry at work, yet it quietly runs the entire show inside you. Every bite of food, every sip of water, every supplement or medication is taken in, broken apart, evaluated and either absorbed or rejected. Your body works constantly, adjusting chemical pathways in response to whatever you take in, whatever you burn and whatever you excrete. Those adjustments shape how young you feel, how strong you stay and how long you live.

People often think youth is something you build on the surface with creams, hair appointments or the occasional bit of Botox, yet the reality is far less glamorous. What makes you feel young comes from the chemistry running inside you, the constant movement of molecules, hormones, enzymes and nutrients keeping your system working as it should. When that internal chemistry is ignored or pushed off balance, the signs you notice are rarely about age; they are usually the result of processes that have been struggling for far longer than you realised.

In reality, you're not just a body, you're a walking chemical lab with billions of reactions happening every second, completely out of sight. Whether those reactions keep you energised or exhausted, strong or brittle, clear-headed or foggy depends on the inputs you control.

When I talk about chemistry as a pillar of regeneration, I'm not talking about abstract science you left behind in school. I'm talking about real things including the choices you make every single day such as:
- What goes in your mouth.
- What goes through your skin.
- What circulates in your blood.

It all causes a reaction.

Here's where I get blunt: most people are flying blind with their chemistry. They throw back a few multivitamins, maybe eat a salad on a Tuesday and hope their internal chemistry sorts itself out. That's not design, that's gambling and is a terrible strategy for staying healthy.

What you want is controlled design. The ability to steer your internal environment like an engineer tweaking a machine. That's what this chapter is about: how to take charge of your chemistry so you can stack the odds in your favour for a very long life.

Here's a thought that might surprise you.

If you want to become a doctor, what A-level do you definitely need? Chemistry. I know, it's unexpected but to begin to study medicine, you can get away without biology but not without chemistry. That should make you think.

Why? Medicine is chemistry in action. Everything from the painkiller you take for a headache to the hormone treatment that saves your bones after menopause, that's chemistry shaping your life. The difference between thriving and barely functioning often comes down to molecules.

The Problem with How We See Chemistry

When most people hear the word "chemistry", they picture a school lab, a Bunsen burner and that one kid who nearly set their sleeve on fire. Or some wild-haired scientist cackling over bubbling green liquid in a glass beaker.

That's the stereotype. The reality though is that chemistry isn't something in a lab, it's inside you. Every second, your body runs a chemical factory, breaking things down, building things up, recycling, detoxing, repairing.

Think about your morning as a whole, from the first sip of coffee that wakes you up as caffeine binds to adenosine receptors in your brain, to the breakfast that becomes a blend of chemical compounds broken down for energy and nutrients, and even the shower gel containing chemicals your skin absorbs, because by the time the clock hits 8am you're already swimming in chemistry, even if you don't often think of it that way.

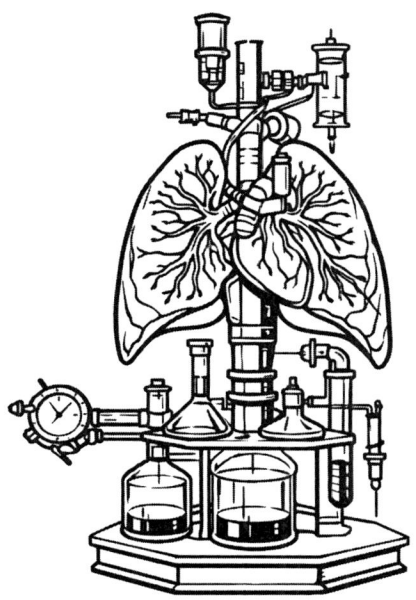

And here's the big question: do you want to leave those reactions to chance, or do you want to run the lab?

Why This Matters

Chemistry isn't neutral, it's either working for you or against you. Ignore it and you open the door to chronic inflammation, hormonal chaos, accelerated ageing and fatigue that no amount of coffee can fix. Take control of it and you unlock energy, resilience and repair at a level most people only dream about.

The good news is that you don't need a PhD to understand enough to make powerful changes. You only need a plan and the willingness to see your body for what it is: a living, breathing chemical system that responds to what you feed it, expose it to and demand from it.

From Ancient Hacks to Modern Mastery

This isn't a new idea, humans have been hacking their chemistry for thousands of years. Long before white coats and pill bottles, ancient civilizations were grinding roots, brewing teas and fermenting plants, all in a quest to control pain, fight infection, or boost vitality.

The first pharmacists weren't in labs, they were in temples, forests and kitchens. Every painkiller in your cabinet today has a family tree stretching back to early experiments.

This chapter will show you how to work with your chemistry, not against it. It will show you how to make better choices about what you consume, check what is actually going on inside your body and use modern science effectively without falling for marketing hype.

Why chemistry matters more than you think.

Modern medicine feels advanced: machines that beep, drugs with names you can't pronounce and robotic surgeries. However, in many ways, our ancestors were wiser than we are. They didn't have MRI scanners or molecular diagrams, yet they understood something most of us have forgotten: the body is part of the earth and what heals us comes from it. Humans have been biohacking chemistry for thousands of years.

They didn't separate food from medicine or mind from body or talk about holistic wellness because life was holistic by default. Wise women, herbalists, healers - they weren't guessing, they were observing patterns for generations, connecting symptoms to seasons, plants to physiology and humans to nature in ways we now pay thousands to relearn.

What matters here isn't history for its own sake. It's that regeneration has always depended on chemistry, whether or not we had the language to describe it.

Pillar 2 - Chemistry: The Invisible War

Take Saint Hildegard of Bingen, a 12th-century Benedictine nun. She wrote extensively about healing with plants, understanding not just what they did for the body but how they affected the soul. Her remedies were rooted in a belief that imbalance in the body reflected imbalance in life, a concept modern science is just rediscovering under the name psychoneuroimmunology.

In modern terms, she was observing how chemistry, environment and nervous system state interact to influence healing.

> *"The earth which sustains humanity must not be injured, it must not be destroyed."*
> Saint Hildegard of Bingen (12th Century)

Before Hildegard, Ayurvedic practitioners in India mapped out entire systems for balancing the body's chemistry using herbs, minerals and food combinations. Traditional Chinese Medicine built theories of energy flow that, when translated, look remarkably like what we now know about circulation and nervous systems.

> *"There are no incurable diseases – only the lack of will. There are no useless herbs – only the lack of knowledge."*
> Avicenna (Ibn Sina, 980–1037)

Did they know about serotonin and dopamine? No and yet they understood how behaviour, food and environment shaped mood and vitality. They knew turmeric reduced swelling long before anyone uttered the word inflammation and they knew bitter herbs aided digestion before we discovered enzymes.

The common thread across all these traditions is simple: change chemistry and you change outcomes.

Contrast that with today: we've got wearable tech, lab diagnostics, supplement aisles that look like candy shops and yet people are more disconnected from their own bodies than ever. Many of us don't even notice thirst signals until we have a headache. Fatigue is normal, bloating is ignored and stress is managed with more caffeine and screen time.

Maybe the question isn't whether ancient people were ignorant. Maybe it's whether we've traded wisdom for convenience.

The Chemistry Thread Through Time

Hippocrates, the Father of Medicine, prescribed willow bark for fever and pain, a practice that evolved into aspirin. In the Islamic Golden Age, Avicenna wrote *The Canon of Medicine*, mapping out remedies from herbs, oils and minerals that shaped medical thinking for 700 years. Galen in Rome created complex botanical formulas that laid the groundwork for pharmacy.

> *"Let food be thy medicine and medicine be thy food."*
> Hippocrates (c. 400 BC)

In China, Shennong, the Divine Farmer, is said to have tasted hundreds of herbs to catalogue their effects, creating the foundation of Traditional Chinese Medicine. In Europe, wise women carried knowledge of healing plants in their heads and hands, treating communities with poultices and teas long before hospitals existed.

Pillar 2 - Chemistry: The Invisible War

> *"The first requirement of a hospital is that it should do the sick no harm."*
> Florence Nightingale (19th Century)

Even hygiene, something we now take for granted, was once revolutionary. Florence Nightingale introduced strict sanitation in military hospitals, slashing infection rates. Ignaz Philipp Semmelweis discovered that washing hands with chlorinated water could save mothers' lives in maternity wards, an idea so radical at the time that his peers mocked him for it. Louis Pasteur later proved what these pioneers suspected, that disease could be carried by invisible agents: germs. His work didn't just change medicine, it changed chemistry itself, leading to antiseptics, vaccines and antibiotics.

> *"The microbes will have the last word."*
> Louis Pasteur (1822–1895)

Pasteur proved what had been invisible for centuries, but the story of medicine didn't start with laboratories or scientific proof. It began in the fields and forests, with people using plants long before they understood the chemistry behind them. Those crude remedies are the roots of the medicines we rely on today.

The Family Tree of Modern Medicine

Morphine didn't appear in a shiny lab out of nowhere. It began as opium, the milky latex from the poppy plant, cultivated as early as 3400 BC by the Sumerians, who called it the *Hul Gil*, the Joy Plant. They didn't know why it worked. They just knew it dulled pain and made suffering tolerable.

The knowledge spread like wildfire: through Egypt, where poppy resin was used in surgical preparations, to Greece, where Hippocrates noted its power, and into the Roman Empire, where Galen used it as a standard for pain control. Fast forward to the early 19th century, when Friedrich Sertürner, a German chemist, isolated the active compound and named it morphine, after Morpheus, the Greek god of dreams. Today, that ancient sap is behind some of the most powerful painkillers in modern medicine.

The same story repeats with aspirin. The ancient Greeks and Native Americans brewed willow bark tea to calm fevers and soothe aches. They didn't talk about salicylic acid, but they knew it worked. In the 1800s, chemists extracted that bitter compound and refined it into acetylsalicylic acid, what we now call aspirin. One of the world's most common medicines, born from tree bark.

Then there is quinine. Long before it became famous as the bite in your gin and tonic, it was extracted from the bark of the cinchona tree and used by indigenous peoples in South America to treat malaria. Later, it saved the lives of explorers and soldiers worldwide. Even now, quinine can ease cramps, so yes, there's more to that tonic than just a splash of sophistication.

It doesn't stop there, Digitalis, a drug for heart failure, comes from foxglove flowers. Penicillin, the world's first antibiotic, was born from mould. Every modern pharmaceutical has roots in nature. Literally.

The point is simple; every pill you take carries a history with it. Modern medicine didn't replace nature, it just bottled it, concentrated it and sometimes forgot the rest of the story.

Regenerative medicine works when we remember that chemistry is not new, it's just been fragmented.

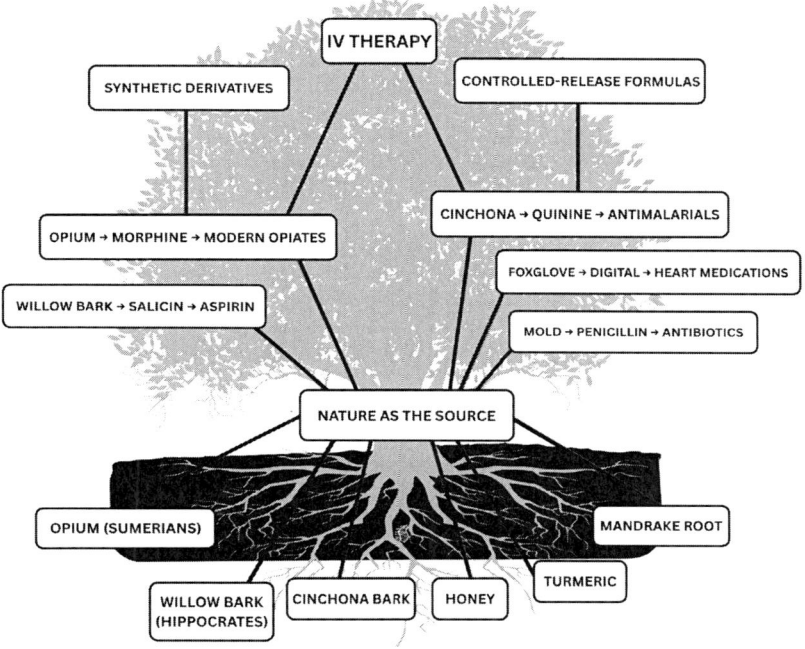

The Modern Problem: Too Much, Too Blind

Today, we're drowning in choice. More protein, more pills, more powders. Scroll Instagram and you'll find "must-have" supplements updated weekly, or walk into a health store and there are so many choices that it can be overwhelming.

Here's where people go wrong: they think more is better. That's not the case, more is definitely not better. Better is better.

Adding random chemicals to your body without understanding what you need, is like throwing spices into a stew without tasting it first. A pinch of salt can transform the dish. Half a jar? Ruined.

Here's the main point, the wrong chemistry can hurt you. Too much iron can lead to inflammation risk or overload vitamin A and you may end up with liver damage. Even safe supplements like B vitamins can cause nerve problems when overdone. This is why it's so important to know your body and understand its needs.

Therefore, it's clear, the goal isn't more, what you need is precision. Consider the best of both worlds: the wisdom of the past and the tools of the present. That means testing before guessing. Targeted changes instead of throwing the whole pharmacy down your throat and using delivery systems that actually work instead of chasing trends.

The rest of this chapter is about doing what the wise women and healers of the past would approve of: restoring balance and supporting vitality but with the advantage of modern diagnostics and delivery systems.

The truth is most of what people blame on "just getting older" isn't fate. It's chemistry, which is something you can influence, if you know how.

Your Internal MOT - Bloods, DNA and Hormones

Ancient healers didn't have today's understanding, but they still checked for signs: they read your pulse and examined your tongue and your eyes. They watched how you moved, how you slept and what your skin looked like, because they knew that the body always gives clues.

Pulse reading and tongue checks were the original biomarkers. Ancient practitioners understood patterns: slow pulse meant energy depletion, a coated tongue suggested digestive issues. Today, we have hundreds of biomarkers and advanced imaging, but the principle hasn't changed: look for clues before the crisis hits. The only difference now is that we can see what's happening at a cellular level, long before symptoms appear due to genetic insights and biomarkers.

Your blood reflects the truth of your internal chemistry and if you ignore it, you may overlook problems you needed to catch early.

Why Guessing is Stupid

Health has nothing to do with chance. It responds to what you monitor and what you change, which means measurement comes first. Supplements aren't bad but without testing, you're throwing darts blindfolded. Even "healthy eaters" often have gaps. Stress, training load and genetics all change your nutrient needs. Guessing is chaos – testing is clarity.

Here's what happens when you play the guessing game:
- You waste money.
- You overload things you don't need.
- You ignore gaps that matter.

Take sodium - too little and your blood pressure crashes, leaving you dizzy and weak. Too much and you're on the fast track to hypertension and heart problems. Or consider calcium - vital for bones but overload can harden your arteries. Balance isn't optional it's the whole game.

Your Health MOT Checklist

Not everything matters. These do:

Blood Work Basics

Why these markers matter:
- **Vitamin D:** Crucial for bone strength, immune defence and mood regulation. Low levels increase risk of fractures and depression.
- **Magnesium:** Supports over 300 enzyme reactions, including muscle function and nervous system

stability. Low magnesium hides behind fatigue, poor sleep and muscle cramps.
- **Iron & Ferritin:** Too little and you're exhausted. Too much and you're damaging organs. Both ends of the spectrum are dangerous.
- **Omega-3 Index:** Low levels drive inflammation and impair brain function. This is one of the easiest wins for longevity.
- **Glucose & HbA1c:** HbA1c is your three-month blood sugar report. If the number is high, your system has been under constant glucose stress and that speeds up ageing in every tissue.
- **CRP:** The silent age accelerator. A normal GP test might flag nothing, but a high-sensitivity CRP can reveal systemic inflammation, one of the biggest predictors of chronic disease.
- **Thyroid Panel:** Your metabolism's thermostat. If this is off, nothing works the way it should.
- **Lipid Profile (cholesterol, LDL, HDL, triglycerides):** Shows how well you process fats and how much strain your cardiovascular system is under.

Hormones
- **Oestrogen, Progesterone, Testosterone:** For mood, muscle and longevity. Menopause and andropause change the game, so track it.
- **Cortisol:** Your stress hormone. High for too long? Welcome to inflammation and burnout.
- **DHEA:** A resilience marker linked to the pace of ageing, influencing energy, recovery, immune function and overall vitality, so it's worth keeping an eye on as the years climb.

Advanced Markers

- **Homocysteine (an amino acid linked to cardiovascular risk):** High levels irritate blood vessels and raise inflammation. Often corrected with B vitamins once tested.
- **DNA Methylation (a marker of biological age):** This measures biological age by looking at chemical markers on your DNA that control how genes switch on and off. A result can show that you are 50 on paper but your cells are behaving like those of someone ten years younger or older.
- **Telomere Length (the protective caps on your chromosomes):** They shorten every time a cell divides and when they become too short, cell ageing accelerates. You can't stop this process, but lifestyle and chemistry choices can slow the rate of shortening.

Genetics: Your Blueprint, Not Your Fate

Why can some people drink three espressos and sleep like a saint, while others get heart palpitations from one latte? Genetics. Your DNA influences how you process caffeine, alcohol, fats, even exercise response.

Your genetic code stays the same throughout your life, yet the way those genes behave is constantly shaped by your habits. This is the essence of epigenetics. It looks at chemical tags that sit on your DNA and act like switches, controlling which genes are active and which stay quiet. These switches respond directly to your lifestyle. Food, stress, sleep, movement, exposure to toxins and even long-term inflammation can all change how your genes express themselves.

Pillar 2 - Chemistry: The Invisible War

You can't rewrite your DNA sequence, but you can influence the environment it sits in. That environment determines whether a gene that promotes repair is switched on, or whether a gene linked to inflammation stays active for longer than it should. This is why two people with the same genetic starting point, including identical twins, can age at completely different speeds and develop very different health outcomes. Epigenetics shows that you aren't stuck with the hand you were dealt. You have the ability to influence how your genes function every day.

In regenerative practice, genetic testing can offer context, but it is not a prerequisite for progress. Most meaningful change happens by improving the environment genes respond to, rather than obsessing over the code itself.

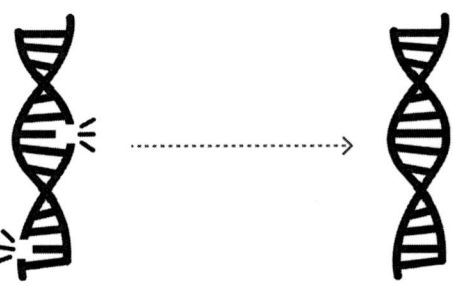

Why BMI Doesn't Tell the Whole Story

Everyone knows their BMI, right? Doctors love it, charts love it but here's the truth: BMI is a blunt tool. It was designed in the 19th century to track population health, not to assess individual fitness. It ignores muscle, bone density and even ethnic differences in body composition. A rugby player can show up as "obese" on the BMI chart while being metabolically healthier than a slim office worker.

What really matters? Chemistry. The internal markers we just covered, blood sugar, inflammation, lipid balance and hormones. These tell you more about your health than a height-weight ratio ever will.

Something few people understand is that your body already has a preferred weight range. This is called your *set point* and it's not a fixed number; it's a range your body works to defend. Drop too far below it and chemistry kicks in. Hunger hormones like ghrelin rise; leptin, which signals fullness, falls and your thyroid may even slow down to conserve energy. The result? Fatigue, cravings and eventually, weight regain. It's not a lack of willpower; it's biology and chemistry doing what they're wired to do, to protect you.

Gain weight and the opposite happens: your metabolism often speeds up to push you back towards that range. It's like your body has an internal thermostat, constantly adjusting to keep you "safe".

This doesn't mean weight management is hopeless, it just means the game isn't always about calories in vs calories out. It's about working with your chemistry, not against it, managing hormones, blood sugar, inflammation and stress so your body feels comfortable at a healthy range. When chemistry is balanced, everything else becomes easier.

No amount of green smoothies will fix a hormone imbalance. Test, don't guess.

How Often Should You Test?

Once a year, minimum. More if you're changing diet, training hard or hitting new life stages. Health isn't static. Your chemistry isn't either.

Testing - a sensible view:
- Annual MOT: Everyone should do this, even if you feel great. Prevention beats cure.
- Quarterly: If you're training hard, recovering from illness, or making major lifestyle changes.
- Life-stage triggers: Pregnancy, menopause and midlife shifts for men all demand extra attention.

Health isn't static, neither is your chemistry. The more your life changes, the more often you should check.

Accessing Tests

You don't need a GP to green-light this. At-home kits can cover most basics and for full panels, private labs are worth the investment, rather than leaving your health to chance.

Hormones - The Master Switches

Hormones aren't background noise. They're the messengers that coordinate energy, metabolism, muscle tone, mood, sleep and even skin health. When you overlook them, you miss the signals that explain why your body is behaving the way it is.

When they're balanced, life feels easier and when they're not, nothing works the way it should.

What Hormones Actually Do

Hormones can talk to each other so when one goes off track, the others often follow. High cortisol from chronic stress can block thyroid conversion, which slows your metabolism. Low oestrogen during menopause affects serotonin, which influences mood. It's a web, not a single wire, that's why chasing one hormone with a single solution rarely works as you have to look at the whole network.

Hormones are messengers: they tell cells what to do and when to do it, like turning on fat-burning, increasing muscle repair, regulating blood sugar or calming inflammation.

Hormones don't run on a fixed setting. They rise and fall during the day and many decline with age, and when they do, the effects are significant. What people call "getting older" is often chemistry changing underneath them.

The Big Players

Oestrogen & Progesterone

These two do far more than affect reproduction. Oestrogen supports bones, the heart, brain function and even collagen for skin. Progesterone calms the nervous system and helps you sleep. When these decline, you don't just get hot flushes, you get metabolic changes, bone loss, mood swings and disrupted sleep.

Testosterone

Everyone needs it. Low testosterone in men means muscle loss, lower energy and poor recovery, high conversion to DHT (a testosterone derivative) is a major factor in male-pattern hair loss. Too little and you feel flat, too much and your hairline pays the price.

Women can also consider testosterone supplementation, under appropriate medical guidance, as it can significantly improve mood, motivation and drive, particularly when traditional HRT has not addressed these symptoms.

Cortisol

The stress hormone. You need it as without cortisol, you wouldn't survive but chronic high levels? They break you down from the inside: muscle loss, belly fat, poor sleep and constant fatigue. Please forget the influencer hacks and magic pills promising to "lower your cortisol", that's marketing, not science. Cortisol balance comes from lifestyle, recovery and addressing stress first.

Insulin

It's having a moment thanks to TikTok and glucose monitors. Influencers love to talk about "glucose spikes", but here's the truth: sugar isn't the only player. Sleep, stress, muscle mass and even meal timing affect blood sugar. Insulin is a storage hormone and when it's working, you burn and store energy efficiently. When your cells stop responding (insulin resistance), you're on the road to fatigue, weight gain and metabolic chaos.

Thyroid Hormones

TSH, T3 and T4 keep metabolism ticking. If your thyroid slows, so does everything else: energy, mood and weight regulation. In the UK however, most routine checks only include TSH. T4 and T3 often aren't tested unless you push for it, and they matter. If you suspect thyroid issues, advocate for yourself or consider private testing.

Menopause: The Chemistry Storm

If you've been told menopause is "just something all women go through the same", you've been lied to. It's not a gentle transition; it's a full-body chemical storm. Oestrogen, progesterone and testosterone all shift and the effects ripple everywhere.

Menopause isn't a single event; it's a phase that can last a decade. Perimenopause starts years before your last period, often without warning. You might still have cycles but symptoms such as brain fog, heavy bleeding and joint pain, are already showing.

Here's what helps: track your symptoms, track your cycle (yes, still) and check your bloods. You're still you, it's the chemistry underneath that's shifting. If your GP doesn't listen, write your symptoms down and take them to the appointment. Facts are hard to ignore.

Hot flushes? Yes. But also:
- Sudden fat gain, especially around the middle.
- Mood swings that feel like someone hijacked your brain.

- Sleep that vanishes just when you need it most.
- Bone density falling faster than you think.
- Libido tanking for no apparent reason.

Then there's the stress. When you don't feel like yourself and when your body feels like an enemy camp, cortisol rises. Chronic stress makes symptoms worse, it's a vicious loop that wrecks confidence and energy.

Menopause is not something to "get through". It's a shift that needs a strategy. That might include lifestyle changes, targeted supplements, or medical options like Hormone Replacement Therapy. (HRT – provides controlled doses of hormones that reduce over time, reinforcing the signals that support sleep, mood, bone strength, metabolism and cognitive clarity. It restores balance rather than attempting to reverse age.) HRT is one of the most researched therapies out there and for many women, it's the difference between surviving and thriving. Is it for everyone? Not always, it depends on individual circumstances.

Know the Clues:

Your body gives early warnings before blood tests do.
- Waking up tired even after a full night's sleep? Thyroid or cortisol could be out of sync.
- Losing hair at the temples? That's often DHT,
- a testosterone derivative, creeping up.
- Cravings and energy crashes mid-afternoon? Insulin may be struggling.
- Anxiety out of nowhere? Low progesterone can trigger it.

Bottom line: If your GP brushes you off, don't settle for it, you deserve better. Find someone who listens, tests properly and works with you on a personalised plan.

Why Testing Matters (and Why It's Not Always Easy)

Practical Reality: In the UK, most GPs will test TSH for thyroid and basic lipids, but full panels are rare unless you push. Testosterone in men is often ignored unless fertility is the issue. Oestrogen and progesterone is almost never checked outside of fertility treatment, down to economics, but it does mean if you want a full picture, you may need private options.

The Men's Midlife Shift (a.k.a. The Midlife Crisis)

Men don't have a menopause moment, but testosterone decline is real. It's called andropause (or even manopause) and it creeps in slowly – less muscle, more belly fat, energy crashes, mood swings and libido fading. That shiny convertible and 25-year-old girlfriend? They won't fix your hormones so you would be better off getting tested and if you need support, use science, not denial.

The Big Truth About Hormones

You can't meditate your way out of a hormone imbalance, nor can you fix it with a green juice or a viral supplement stack. Supplements can help but they're tools, not magic bullets. The foundation is testing, smart lifestyle choices and personalised interventions. Balance your hormones and the rest becomes easier, ignore them and you'll keep wondering why everything feels like a fight.

Hormone Myths That Need To Disappear

Myth 1: "Ashwagandha will fix your stress."
Reality: It might take the edge off, but it won't cancel out a high-pressure job, no sleep and four double espressos. Supplements work best on top of solid habits, not instead of them.

Myth 2: "Lion's Mane coffee = focus unlocked."
Reality: Mushroom powders won't rewire your brain overnight. The evidence is promising for nerve health but if your diet is junk and you're running on fumes, no latte will save you.

Myth 3: "Berberine is nature's Ozempic."
Reality: Berberine can support blood sugar control but it's not a miracle fat-loss pill. If it was, pharmacies would have empty shelves.

Myth 4: "Anti-bloat powders will give you a flat stomach."
Reality: Most of these are overpriced laxatives in pretty jars. Bloating usually means intestinal system imbalance or hormonal shifts. Powders don't fix root causes.

Myth 5: "Supplements solve everything."
Reality: They can support but they're not magic in capsules. Test first, then decide what you actually need. Do your research thoroughly – not just from Dave down the pub whose mum swears by them or Chantell on Instagram with 5 million followers being paid to create the post.

My Hormone Guide:

- Test before you guess. Symptoms point you in the right direction, but bloods confirm.
- Look at trends, rather than snapshots. One test on a bad day doesn't define you.
- Balance first, optimise second. Fix the basics before chasing enhancements.
- Lifestyle is chemistry: sleep, stress, food and training shape your hormonal health.
- Use science when you need it. HRT, TRT, peptides, they're tools, not taboos.

The Chemistry Of What You Eat

Most people treat food like petrol for a car. Fill up, burn it off, job done, but although your body is a physics engine, it's also a living lab. Every bite you take sends chemical instructions, some switch on repair, balance and energy, while others stoke inflammation, age your cells and wreck your hormones.

Food as Chemistry, Not Calories

Forget "eat less, move more". If it worked, everyone would be lean and full of energy. Your body doesn't run on maths; it runs on chemical reactions.

Eat protein and you trigger muscle repair and release hormones that help you feel satisfied. Eat fibre and you feed gut bacteria that create anti-inflammatory compounds. Eat ultra-processed junk and you flood your system with additives, trans fats and sugar that spikes insulin and keeps your cells in a state of chaos.

Food isn't just fuel, it's information. Good information builds resilience – bad information breaks it.

Pillar 2 - Chemistry: The Invisible War

Your plate is a control panel. Every choice sends signals that can either keep your system stable or throw it into chaos. Eat high-sugar, low-fibre food and you don't just "gain weight", you set off a chain reaction: blood glucose spikes, insulin floods your system, energy crashes and cravings roar back stronger. Do that repeatedly and you're not just tired, you're on the fast track to insulin resistance.

On the flip side, when you combine protein, healthy fats and fibre, you keep blood sugar stable and hormones like leptin and ghrelin, the ones that control hunger and satiety, working in your favour. That's chemistry you can control every time you pick up a fork.

Why Inflammation Matters

Inflammation is your body's defence system, but when it never switches off, it becomes your biggest foe. Chronic low-grade inflammation accelerates ageing, weakens immunity, damages joints and fogs your brain. It also drives insulin resistance and hormone disruption.

What fuels this fire?
- Processed seed oils like sunflower and soybean oil in cheap snacks and fast food
- Ultra-processed carbohydrates
- Excess sugar in everything from "healthy" granola to plant-based bars
- Stress and lack of sleep (yes, lifestyle is chemistry too)

Know Your Signals: If you're feeling constantly tired, that could point to blood sugar instability or low iron. Persistent brain fog is often tied to low omega-3 intake or chronic inflammation. While craving sugar all day could be sleep debt and a cortisol imbalance might be to blame as much as diet.

You won't always feel inflammation, but it shows in blood work, in joint pain, in slow recovery, in the creeping sense of exhaustion you blame on age.

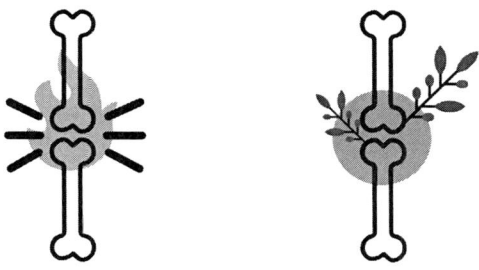

Smart Chemistry Note: When More Pills Make Things Worse

Here is something most people do not consider. Low oestrogen during perimenopause and menopause heightens the sensitivity of pain receptors, which means headaches, joint aches and muscle pain register more strongly. Many women turn to increasing doses of pain medication because the discomfort feels sharper and more persistent.

However, medication that pushes inflammation down without addressing the cause can place stress on the gut and digestion. Non-steroidal anti-inflammatory drugs (such as ibuprofen) and stronger painkillers can irritate the stomach lining, slow bowel movements and contribute to bloating, which is already more common as hormone levels fall. The better approach is to steady the chemistry that drives the pain rather than only silencing the signal. Nutrition, stress control and targeted medical support can all reduce inflammation at its source.

Powerful Anti-Inflammatory Chemistry

Inflammation rises when the body deals with ongoing stress, poor sleep, toxins or unstable blood sugar. Persistent inflammation places pressure on the systems responsible for repair and regeneration. Certain nutrients support the pathways that regulate this response and ease the load on those systems. These have the strongest evidence:

- **Omega-3 fats**: Found in salmon, sardines and other oily fish, as well as nuts and seeds. These fats help reduce inflammation because the body uses them to repair membranes and calm the chemical signals that drive pain and swelling.
- **Polyphenols**: Found in berries, dark chocolate and colourful plants. These compounds neutralise free radicals and reduce oxidative stress, which lowers the chemical signals that drive inflammation.
- **Spices**: Turmeric (curcumin), ginger and cinnamon. These ingredients block key enzymes involved in the inflammatory response and help moderate pain and swelling.
- **Olive oil**: Rich in monounsaturated fats and antioxidants. It reduces inflammatory signalling in blood vessels and supports metabolic stability.
- **Green tea**: Packed with catechins. These compounds reduce oxidative stress, support detoxification pathways and help calm low-grade inflammation.

Before redesigning your entire diet, check the basics. Blood tests for HbA1c, a full lipid panel, vitamin D, ferritin and CRP provide a clear picture of how your internal chemistry is functioning. These numbers guide your choices and enable you to amend your diet more efficiently.

A simple rule helps. When most of the food on the plate is beige, your chemistry carries the strain.

Diet Trends That Waste Your Time (and What Actually Works)

The idea of food as medicine isn't new. Hippocrates said it centuries ago: *"Let food be thy medicine and medicine be thy food."* Today, biochemistry explains why he was right. The phytonutrients in plants, the amino acids in protein, the healthy fats in olive oil, they don't just feed you. They act as signalling molecules, flipping genetic switches, calming inflammation and supporting repair.

Greens Powders
Why they sound good: They contain powdered vegetables, vitamins and minerals, so the pitch is that you get your daily greens in one scoop.

Why that's not the full story: Processing strips away fibre and many bioactive compounds that protect your intestinal system and reduce inflammation.

What to do instead: Eat real plants in a variety of colours. Fibre isn't optional; it's a chemical signal your gut microbiome needs to reduce inflammation and support hormone balance.

Celery Juice Detox

Why it sounds good: Celery contains water, minerals and antioxidants. Claims suggest it "alkalises" your body and supports detoxification.

Reality check: Your body detoxes 24/7 through your liver, kidneys and lungs. No single juice "flushes toxins". Plus can you imagine how awful this tastes?

What to do instead: Support your liver with what it needs: hydration, protein for amino acids that fuel detox enzymes and plenty of colourful vegetables for antioxidants.

Chlorophyll Water

Why it sounds good: Chlorophyll is in green plants and plants are healthy, so drinking it must be too, right? Claims link it to improved skin, energy and "oxygenation".

Reality check: Oral chlorophyll doesn't behave like the chlorophyll in plants. You're not photosynthesising; you're paying for green dye in fancy packaging.

What to do instead: Eat real greens like spinach and rocket: they give you chlorophyll plus iron, magnesium and polyphenols that actually benefit your cells.

Can you see the trend there? It's not rocket science, but there should be rocket in your salad!

Glucose Hacks

Why it sounds good: Continuous glucose monitors show real-time sugar spikes. Lower spikes = better health. It's logical.

Reality check: Glucose response isn't just about food, it's about sleep, stress, hydration and muscle activity. You can eat "perfectly" and still see spikes if you're sleep-deprived or stressed.

What to do instead: Build muscle (it's your biggest glucose sink), prioritise sleep and balance meals with protein and fibre. That's what stabilises blood sugar long-term, not vinegar shots.

Alkaline Diets
Why it sounds good: Disease thrives in an "acidic" environment, so eating alkaline foods must prevent it.

Reality check: Your body tightly regulates blood pH between 7.35 and 7.45. If food could change that, you'd be in intensive care.

What to do instead: Focus on nutrient density. Alkaline diets work because they accidentally tell you to eat vegetables and avoid processed junk, so do that without the fake science.

My Quick Framework for Eating with Chemistry in Mind:
- Build meals around quality protein and a rainbow of plants.
- Cut ultra-processed oils and sugar as they're inflammation accelerators.
- Add colour to your plate: pigments in berries, greens and spices are natural anti-inflammatory compounds.
- Time your meals to avoid constant grazing.

Give your insulin levels room to breathe.

Supplements That Actually Make Sense

Supplements are tools and are worth considering when testing shows gaps, or when life makes perfection impossible:
- **Vitamin D:** Most of us in the UK are low, especially in winter.
- **Omega-3**: If you're not eating oily fish twice a week, supplement it.
- **Collagen + Vitamin C:** Supports joint health and skin structure as natural production declines. Without vitamin C the collagen is not effective. Also vitamin C promotes stem cell functions and release.
- **Vitamin B:** there are lots of coenzymes which need it for metabolism regeneration. One of the most important vitamins in the body.
- **Magnesium:** Crucial for energy, recovery and sleep.
- **Peptides and exosomes:** These aren't pills, they're cutting-edge regenerative therapies I use in clinic. More on that later.

The golden rule is test first and check for quality, don't buy everything an influencer waves in your face.

My Chemistry Guide for Eating
- If it comes in a packet with more than five ingredients, leave it.
- If it looks beige and lifeless, so will you.
- Protein isn't a trend; it's a requirement.
- Plants aren't just garnish; they're chemistry labs in disguise.
- Hydrate like an adult: water first, hype drinks later.

I appreciate that not everyone has the financial ability to go private for testing or medical treatments, so a lot of what I've talked about in this chapter you can do quite simply and at low cost. But, in order to live a longer and healthy life and to regenerate your body, you must see it as a long-term investment.

Advanced Chemistry - Beyond Food And Pills

Once you've mastered the basics: balanced nutrition, smart movement and stress control, here's where things get interesting. Think of this as Formula 1 for your biology. The foundations keep the engine running but advanced chemistry is where we push performance, resilience and recovery to the next level.

This isn't biohacking in the TikTok sense of butter coffee and ice baths. It's precision medicine using science and engineering to give your body the signals it needs to repair, regenerate and perform at its best.

Why Pills Alone Aren't Enough

As I said in the last chapter, supplements matter. They can provide essential nutrients that most of us don't get enough of through food alone. Popping capsules isn't the most efficient way to deliver certain compounds into your system, as oral supplements face barriers, stomach acid, gut absorption and competition with other nutrients. Even with high-quality products, only a fraction of the active ingredients reach your bloodstream.

That's why advanced chemistry doesn't replace basic supplementation, it builds on it. Once the foundations are in place, we move to delivery systems and compounds that work faster, smarter and deeper.

Important Note

The substances discussed in this section are included for educational purposes only and to reflect current areas of clinical and scientific interest within regenerative medicine. Their inclusion does not constitute endorsement, recommendation, or general suitability. Access to peptides and related therapies sits within regulated medical practice and requires appropriate clinical assessment, prescribing authority, and professional supervision. Any use should be guided by a qualified clinician and based on an individual health evaluation, current evidence, and applicable regulatory frameworks.

A few of the most promising new treatments:

BPC-157
Known as the "body protection compound", it supports gut health, joint repair and soft tissue healing. Athletes use it for faster recovery after injuries.

Thymosin Beta-4
Plays a role in immune modulation and tissue repair, making it valuable for resilience and recovery.

CJC-1295 and Ipamorelin
These peptides stimulate your own growth hormone release, supporting muscle maintenance, fat metabolism and recovery, without the risks associated with synthetic HGH.

Peptides are small chains of amino acids that act as chemical signals, guiding repair, regeneration and immune responses. Their role in recovery and longevity is promising, although research continues to expand. This is why they appear in injury rehabilitation and post-surgical care.

Peptides are an active area of research in regenerative medicine because they can guide repair, immunity and cellular communication in a targeted way. Access sits within clinical care rather than over-the-counter products, with dosing and safety monitored by a medical professional. My own use of them takes place only in controlled settings and only after a full assessment of the person's health profile.

Do your research and find a reputable clinician if you want to look further into this.

Exosomes: Messaging at a Cellular Level

Exosomes are microscopic vesicles that carry proteins, RNA and other signals between cells and they are central to the way tissues coordinate repair and regulation. Research into their use in regenerative medicine is progressing but most of the work remains in laboratories and early human studies rather than routine treatment. Their potential is promising, yet the science is still in motion.

Because of this, exosome-based therapies require regulated sources, strict protocols and expert oversight. They are not available through simple clinics and anyone exploring this field should rely on up-to-date scientific guidance rather than commercial claims.

IV Therapy: Chemistry, Direct to Your Cells – As Close As We Can Get

Most oral nutrients lose a large percentage of their potency before reaching your bloodstream. This is because of something called first-pass metabolism, where your digestive system and liver break down a significant amount of what you take in. For example, high-dose vitamin C taken orally hits an absorption ceiling at around 200 mg per dose. IV delivery can safely provide 10 to 20 grams, which is why it's used clinically to support immunity and recovery.

IV therapy bypasses the digestive tract and delivers nutrients directly into your bloodstream for 100% bioavailability and immediate cellular uptake.

Regen 365

That's why I designed **Regen 365**, to support the body at its most fundamental level: cellular energy. When the body is under stress from surgery, illness, injury, or prolonged fatigue, energy production drops long before symptoms fully appear. Regen 365 focuses on restoring that internal environment so the body can repair, recover and function more effectively.

Unlike oral supplements, IV therapy bypasses digestion and delivers nutrients straight into the bloodstream. This means cells receive what they need immediately, without losses from absorption limits or gut processing.

In simple terms, Regen 365 is about recharging the systems that keep you alive and resilient, starting at the cellular level.

Pillar 2 - Chemistry: The Invisible War

What Regen 365 Is Designed to Support

The Three Core Energy Systems

Energy System	What It Supports	Why It Matters
Cellular Fuel Entry	Turns nutrients into usable cellular energy	Without this step, energy production never fully switches on
Energy Cycling	Keeps energy production steady and sustainable	Prevents crashes, fatigue and metabolic slowdown
Cellular Power Output	Produces ATP, the body's energy currency	ATP fuels repair, movement, immunity and cognition

These systems work together to restore cellular energy rather than forcing stimulation.

The Six Regenerative Systems Regen 365 Supports

System	Primary Benefit
Nervous System	Supports nerve function, focus and resilience
Muscles & Joints	Assists tissue repair and recovery
Immune Balance	Helps regulate inflammation and defence
Circulation	Supports oxygen and nutrient delivery
Detox Pathways	Assists cellular clean-up processes
Genetic Repair	Supports DNA maintenance and longevity pathways

Rather than targeting one symptom, Regen 365 works across systems, creating a more supportive internal environment for healing.

Key Nutrients and Their Roles

Nutrient Group	Role in the Body
B Vitamins	Drive cellular energy production
Vitamin C	Supports tissue repair and immune defence
Amino Acids	Provide building blocks for repair
Minerals	Support nerve signalling and metabolism

These are not exotic substances. They are familiar nutrients delivered in the right form, at the right concentration, in the right way.

When Regen 365 Is Used

Situation	Intended Support
Pre-procedure	Prepares the body for stress and recovery
Post-procedure	Supports repair and energy restoration
Regenerative care	Enhances recovery environments
Long-term vitality	Maintains energy and cellular function

Regen 365 is not a replacement for nutrition, movement or sleep. It is a supportive intervention designed to help the body do what it already knows how to do.

Pillar 2 - Chemistry: The Invisible War

Why IV Delivery Makes the Difference

Most oral supplements never reach full effectiveness due to digestive breakdown and absorption limits. IV delivery avoids this entirely, allowing nutrients to reach cells directly and immediately.

For people looking to make a **measurable change at the cellular level**, delivery matters as much as content.

A Note on Safety and Oversight - Regen 365 is delivered within a clinical setting using established medical protocols. It is designed as an adjunct to care, not a shortcut or substitute for lifestyle foundations.

The Science of Negative Ions

Every chemical reaction in your body relies on the movement of ions. These carry an electrical charge influencing how cells take in nutrients, release energy, repair themselves and communicate. Without ions the chemistry slows, with the right balance, reactions can run smoothly.

What ions are, in simple terms

An ion is simply an atom or molecule that carries a charge because it has gained or lost an electron. When it picks up an extra electron it becomes negatively charged, and when it gives one up it becomes positively charged. Your body relies on these charged particles every second to fire nerves, contract muscles, move fluids, and keep chemical reactions running smoothly.

Why ions matter for your chemistry

Ions create tiny electrical differences across each cell membrane. These differences act as signals that control how nutrients enter a cell, how energy is produced and how repair processes switch on after stress. When these voltage patterns are steady, chemistry flows with precision but if they drift, reactions slow, energy becomes harder to produce and inflammation rises.

Negative ions - why they matter

Negative ions are molecules carrying spare electrons. Those electrons help the body manage the daily wear created by stress, pollution, poor sleep and normal metabolism. When the body has more to clear than it can manage, oxidative stress builds and this leads to:
- higher inflammation
- slower recovery
- tired, inefficient cells

Spare electrons help ease that strain and steady the reactions that keep your chemistry balanced.

Where negative ions come from

Negative ions occur naturally in places where air or water is constantly moving. Coastlines, forests, waterfalls and open outdoor spaces produce air rich in spare electrons. You feel this as fresher air or easier breathing but underneath that sensation is chemistry working with less friction.

The modern ion gap

The majority of us spend our time in electrically "flat" environments. Indoor air systems reduce natural ions, synthetic materials block natural discharge and device-heavy spaces add electrical load without restoring electrons. None of this causes illness directly, yet it increases the effort your body needs to stay stable.

What the research shows

Studies link negative-ion exposure with improvements in:
- inflammatory markers
- sleep rhythm regulation
- heart rate variability
- perceived stress
- overall energy

When electrons are available, chemical pressure drops and cells work with more ease.

Why this helps your chemistry work better

Spare electrons from negative ions support the reactions that keep your internal chemistry steady. When oxidative stress falls, nutrients such as omega-3 fats and polyphenols work more effectively, antioxidants have a clearer path and hormonal signals regain precision. Negative ions are not a fix on their own. They simply reduce friction inside the system so the body can function with greater ease.

Negative ions help reduce the chemical pressure your body carries each day, yet your environment still plays a major part in how easily those electrons reach you. Grounding is the simplest route to restoring that connection and it can be built into ordinary life with almost no effort.

The Pod - Chemistry Meets Physics

Think about how you treat your phone. If the charger slowed to a crawl and gave you a ten per cent boost after hours of waiting, you would replace it without hesitation, because you know there is a faster, more efficient way to deliver power. The body deserves the same consideration. It performs at a higher level when energy and nutrients reach it through an optimised pathway rather than relying entirely on the gut, which can be slow, inconsistent and easily disrupted.

Modern physics allows us to support that process. When heat, pressure and controlled frequency shape the way compounds move through the body, absorption improves and delivery becomes more reliable. This is where physics enhances chemistry, helping essential compounds reach the tissues where they make the greatest difference.

This principle sits at the heart of the Regen PhD Pod and understanding it makes the purpose of the system far clearer. The way something is delivered often determines the impact it can have, and the body responds well when the pathway is upgraded rather than left to its own limitations.

Why Delivery Matters

Your body is a marvel of engineering but it's selective: it decides what gets in, how fast and where it goes. Most supplements rely on digestion, which is effective but not always consistent. Factors like stress, age and stomach health can all affect uptake.

This is current biology and it means we have an opportunity: improve the environment in which nutrients are delivered, and you improve the results. The Regen PhD Pod isn't here to replace what you're already doing, it's here to make it work even better.

The Physics-Chemistry Partnership

The breakthrough is simple. Physics can enhance chemistry when the body is placed in the right state. Instead of fighting through the natural filters that slow absorption, we work with them. Sound, heat, light, magnetic vibration and targeted sensory stimulation shift the body into a receptive mode, creating conditions where nutrients and therapeutic compounds can move with far greater ease.
- **Heat** widens blood vessels and increases circulation, creating a faster, cleaner route for nutrients to travel while priming cells to receive what they are given.
- **Vibration** supports lymphatic movement and cellular exchange, helping waste move out while drawing beneficial compounds in.

- **Light**, especially in specific wavelengths, influences mitochondrial activity, nudging cells to produce more energy and respond more effectively to incoming support.
- **Sound**, when delivered at tuned frequencies, encourages nervous system regulation and helps shift the body out of stress patterns that make absorption less efficient.
- **Magnetic vibration** interacts with the electrical activity of cells, supporting ion movement and helping tissues regain their natural signalling rhythms.

Skin absorption becomes far more effective when these conditions are combined, because the body is already primed for movement, exchange and repair. When physics creates the right state and chemistry provides the right compounds, the result is synergy. Multiple systems work together rather than in isolation, supporting recovery, repair and resilience at a deeper level.

Aromatherapy: Ancient Chemistry, Modern Science

As I mentioned earlier in the chapter, before we had pills, we had plants. Long before the word "aromatherapy" existed, ancient cultures were using aromatic oils and herbs as part of medicine and ritual. The Egyptians embalmed their dead with myrrh and frankincense, two resins with antimicrobial properties still studied today. Greek physicians, including Hippocrates, wrote about using thyme, rosemary and lavender for respiratory and stress-related ailments. In Ayurveda, sandalwood and tulsi (holy basil) were prescribed to calm the mind and strengthen the body. Even the Romans added aromatic herbs to their famous baths because they understood the restorative effects of scent and warmth.

These weren't random choices, they were chemistry experiments and while our ancestors didn't know about neurotransmitters or volatile compounds, they understood the outcome: certain aromas made people calmer, more focused, more resilient.

Today, we know why it works. Aromatic compounds travel through the nose to the olfactory bulb, which connects directly to the limbic system, the part of the brain that controls emotion, memory and stress response. Unlike most substances, they don't need to pass through digestion or the bloodstream first. That means scent is one of the fastest ways to influence the nervous system. Inhalation can modulate neurotransmitters like serotonin and GABA (Gamma-Aminobutyric Acid), your brain's natural calming signal. GABA acts like a brake on nerve activity, reducing stress and promoting relaxation. Some compounds even interact with ion channels and receptors involved in pain perception.

This makes aromatherapy biochemistry delivered by breath. A chemical intervention that's been in use for thousands of years. What the ancients did by instinct, we now understand at the molecular level.

In the Pod, aromatherapy is a functional part of the system. Each scent is chosen for a purpose, with compounds that work synergistically with heat and transdermal nutrients:

- **Coffee:** Stimulates the nervous system, sharpens alertness and enhances focus through compounds like caffeine and chlorogenic acids.
- **Lavender:** High in linalool and linalyl acetate, shown to calm anxiety and promote better sleep by activating GABA pathways.
- **Green Tea:** Contains catechins and theanine, linked to antioxidant effects and a state of calm alertness.
- **Eucalyptus:** Rich in eucalyptol, a terpene that reduces inflammation and supports respiratory function.
- **Aloe:** Known for its soothing, skin-repairing polysaccharides, aiding hydration and tissue recovery.

This is chemistry working through multiple channels: olfactory, dermal and neurological, creating a full-body reset that goes far beyond mood. The ancients used oils and herbs because they worked. We're using the same principles but with precision and science behind every choice.

What This Means for Your Future

The Pod is more than a wellness tool; it's a glimpse into what health will look like in the next decade. It will have smarter delivery systems, personalised protocols that adapt to your unique chemistry and integrated therapies that work with your biology instead of against it.

We've spent decades asking, "What should I take?" The next question is, "How do I make it work better?" That's what this technology answers.

At the time of writing we're only at the beginning. Imagine Pod sessions tailored to your blood biomarkers, delivering compounds in exactly the dose your cells need. Imagine AI-driven programmes that adjust based on your stress levels, recovery metrics and even your mood.

The future of longevity won't be about adding more, it will be about making every input count.

When chemistry and physics combine, that future moves from theory to reality.

Real-life example

Sarah, 48, came to me for an MRI following a series of joint problems. After a consultation it came out that she had been battling fatigue, brain fog and joint pain for over two years. She'd already seen her GP and even had a full blood panel done privately but the results were never joined up into a clear plan. When she came to us, we combined those findings with our own advanced testing to see the bigger picture.

The showed what was actually happening: chronic inflammation, low vitamin D and sluggish mitochondrial function. We started with targeted IV therapy to restore key nutrients and support her energy systems. Within weeks, her fatigue began to lift. Then came peptides, BPC-157 for gut healing and CJC-1295 to naturally boost growth hormone release. These were precision tools given to her based on data.

Now, six months on, Sarah isn't just symptom-free, she feels stronger and sharper than she has in years. She's excited for the next phase, which will include Pod sessions to push her recovery and resilience even further. That's the power of advanced chemistry when it's applied intelligently and monitored properly.

The Big Picture

This is biohacking done properly, with science, precision, safety and strategies that are designed to last. This is about engineering your body to perform better for longer. Advanced chemistry gives us tools that didn't exist a decade ago, tools that move us from survival to optimisation.

Where is this heading? Toward AI-driven health plans, nano-tech that delivers compounds cell by cell and gene therapies that could slow ageing at its root. Advanced chemistry today will look basic in ten years but right now, it's the most powerful longevity toolkit we've ever had.

If you're wondering where to start, here's my framework:
- **Tier 1:** The basics: nutrition, movement, foundational supplements.
- **Tier 2:** Precision, IV therapy and peptides based on personal data.
- **Tier 3:** Elite optimisation, exosomes, Pod sessions and advanced regenerative protocols.

You don't have to master every tier before moving up. You can start where it makes the most sense for your health and your goals. It's worth mentioning though that when these layers work together, the results are exponential.

If you're serious about staying strong, resilient and biologically younger for longer, this is where you start thinking like an engineer, not a gambler.

The Future of Chemistry

Everything we've covered in this chapter is proven and practical – it's what you can do right now to keep your chemistry working for you. What about the future though? That's a different game. We're moving towards a world where we don't just manage decline, we actively repair and even reprogramme the body. If chemistry is today, biotechnology is tomorrow.

The Next Frontier
For centuries, we've worked with what nature gave us: food, herbs, supplements, drugs. Then we learned how to tweak molecules and deliver them more effectively. Now we're stepping into a world where we can rewrite the body's operating system.

Stem Cells:
Stem cells are often described as the master builders of the body because they have the capacity to develop into many different types of tissue. The story is more nuanced when you look at the specific cells used in most regenerative therapies. Mesenchymal Stem Cells, now more accurately described as Medicinal Signalling Cells (MSC), do far more

than attempt to replace damaged tissue. Their primary role is communication. They release signals that guide repair, calm inflammation and influence how neighbouring cells respond to injury or stress.

Current research is exploring their potential to support joint repair, encourage regeneration in heart tissue and provide help in certain neurological conditions. The promise is not limited to slowing the effects of ageing. The real possibility lies in supporting the body's ability to repair what time has already altered.

Peptides:
If vitamins are the building blocks, peptides are the foremen on the construction site. These short chains of amino acids act as signalling molecules, instructing your body to do what it's already designed to do: repair, regenerate and maintain balance.

Ageing is, in many ways, a signalling problem. The hardware still works but the messages become weaker or distorted. Peptides restore those signals, turning on pathways that promote healing and vitality.

Early evidence suggests they could support recovery after surgery, help tissues respond more effectively to stress and perhaps even shift long-term patterns of damage. This positions peptides as one of the most intriguing developments in regenerative science, a field where progress is rapid and the potential is far from fully realised. Anyone exploring them today is stepping into territory that will almost certainly shape the next decade of medical innovation.

Exosomes:
If stem cells are builders, exosomes are the blueprints and messengers. These microscopic vehicles carry instructions between cells, telling them how to repair, grow, or calm inflammation. Clinics are already using exosome therapy for injury recovery and skin rejuvenation. Early research suggests potential for neurodegenerative diseases, immune regulation and metabolic health.

Genetic Editing:
CRISPR technology has turned the dream of gene editing into reality. It allows scientists to "cut and paste" sections of DNA, switching off harmful genes or activating protective ones. Imagine a future where hereditary risks for diseases like Alzheimer's or certain cancers could be silenced before they ever surface. This isn't 50 years away; the trials have already started.

Epigenetic Reprogramming:
Beyond editing genes, scientists are finding ways to reprogramme the signals that control ageing. Epigenetic "switches" determine whether your cells act young or old. Resetting those switches could mean rejuvenating tissues without replacing them.

All of this is coming faster than most people realise. Biotech is extending health spans, keeping your brain sharp, your body strong and your chemistry balanced for decades longer than previous generations.

What This Means for You
Should you wait for the future? No. Here's the truth: these breakthroughs will only work best in a body that's ready for

them. That means the choices you make today matter more than ever. Balanced hormones, low inflammation and strong mitochondria: these are the foundations that will make you a candidate for advanced therapies when they arrive.

Think of it this way: biotech is the next operating system but if your hardware is broken, the upgrade won't run.

The work you've done so far in understanding your chemistry, improving your nutrition, managing hormones and testing and adjusting, isn't a hack - it's preparation. You're building resilience now so you can take advantage of what's next.

The Bottom Line
The future of health isn't about luck. It's about design and the best time to start designing is now.

You're not hacking your health. You're engineering it, one smart chemical choice at a time.

Your Practical Toolkit

Theory is great. Understanding why chemistry matters gives you power to act but action creates results. This toolkit pulls everything you've learned into clear, practical steps. These are science-backed strategies you can start today.

Your goal isn't perfection. It's consistency. Small, smart changes build the chemistry that keeps you young, strong and full of energy.

1. Your Annual MOT Checklist

Think of this as your yearly service. A few simple tests give you the data you need to track health before symptoms show up.

The Essentials (Start Here):
- ☐ **Vitamin D -** Checks your immune and bone health.
- ☐ **Iron & Ferritin -** Shows energy status and risks from overload.
- ☐ **Magnesium -** Often overlooked but critical for energy and nerve function.

- ☐ **Glucose & HbA1c -** Spot blood sugar issues early.
- ☐ **Lipid Profile -** Cholesterol plus ratios for heart health.
- ☐ **CRP (C-Reactive Protein) -** A measure of hidden inflammation.
- ☐ **Ask your GP for Vitamin D, HbA1c, iron studies and basic thyroid. These are often covered if you have symptoms or risk factors. Thyroid Panel (TSH, T3, T4)** is your metabolic control switch, showing how effectively your body manages glucose over the previous three months.

Advanced (Worth Considering):
- ☐ Hormones (oestrogen, progesterone, testosterone, cortisol)
- ☐ Omega-3 Index
- ☐ Homocysteine
- ☐ DNA Methylation & Biological Age
- ☐ Telomere Length

How to Get These Tests:
- ☐ **GP/NHS:** Note – some may not be available and will have to be requested through private clinics.
- ☐ **Private Clinics:** For full panels, including hormones and advanced markers, private labs like Medichecks or Thriva in the UK offer home kits with finger-prick or venous samples.
- ☐ **In-Clinic:** If you want full interpretation and targeted action plans, book a consultation with a clinician who understands longevity and functional health.

Pro Tips:
- ☐ Test after fasting, first thing in the morning.
- ☐ Skip heavy exercise the day before for accurate cortisol and thyroid results.
- ☐ Re-test annually, or every 6 months if making big changes.

2. Sample Anti-Inflammatory Food Plan

Sample 1

Inflammation is the chemistry that ages you fastest. Food is your most powerful lever to calm it down. Here's a simple one-day example.

Breakfast:
Overnight oats with berries, chia seeds and a handful of walnuts.

Why it works: Fibre feeds your gut microbiome; berries deliver polyphenols; walnuts supply omega-3 fats.

Lunch:
Salmon fillet, quinoa and mixed greens with olive oil.

Why it works: Protein for repair; omega-3s for anti-inflammatory effect; olive oil adds antioxidants.

Snacks:
Green tea, dark chocolate (85%+ cocoa) and a small handful of almonds.

Why it works: Catechins fight oxidative stress; magnesium in dark chocolate supports recovery.

Dinner:
Herb-roasted chicken (or tofu) with garlic, greens, and roasted sweet potato.

Why it works: Garlic supports immune and vascular health; greens aid detox pathways; sweet potato provides slow-release carbohydrates and beta-carotene.

Rule of thumb: If your plate looks beige, your chemistry is crying.

Sample 2

Breakfast:
Avocado toast on rye + poached eggs + a side of blueberries.

Why it works: Healthy fats stabilize blood sugar; eggs for protein and choline; blueberries for antioxidants.

Mid-Morning:
Green tea + 30g mixed nuts.

Why it works: Catechins fight oxidative stress; nuts add magnesium and omega-3s.

Lunch:
Grilled salmon salad with olive oil, mixed greens, cherry tomatoes and pumpkin seeds.

Why it works: Omega-3s lower inflammation; greens feed intestinal health; seeds provide zinc.

Snack:
Hummus with cucumber and carrot sticks.

Why it works: Plant fibre + polyphenols to keep blood sugar stable.

Dinner:
Turmeric and ginger-spiced chicken (or tofu) with roasted sweet potato and steamed broccoli.

Why it works: Curcumin and gingerols calm inflammation; sweet potato for beta-carotene; broccoli for sulforaphane detox power.

Evening Wind-Down:
Chamomile tea + 2 squares of 85% cocoa dark chocolate.

Why it works: Relaxation compounds + magnesium for recovery.

Principle: Colour = antioxidants. Beige = trouble.

Pillar 2 - Chemistry: The Invisible War

3. Supplement Matrix

Supplements aren't magic bullets, but they can bridge gaps when life isn't perfect. Here's what matters most:

Nutrient	Why It Matters	When to Consider
Vitamin D	Immunity, bone health, hormone support	If levels test low or in winter months
Omega-3 (EPA/DHA)	Reduces inflammation, supports brain health	If you rarely eat oily fish
Magnesium	Energy production, recovery, sleep	If stressed, fatigued, or poor-quality sleep
Collagen	Joint and skin structure	Ageing, active lifestyle, or injury recovery
Peptides & Exosomes	Advanced regenerative support	In-clinic only; not DIY

Golden rule: Test first as guessing wastes money and time. Quality matters more than quantity.

4. Everyday Chemistry Hacks

These are small, easy wins you can repeat daily. Habits that nudge your chemistry in the right direction:
- **Start hydrated:** Dehydration mimics fatigue and slows cellular repair.
- **Prioritise sleep:** 7–9 hours restores cortisol balance and growth hormone release.
- **Ground yourself:** Barefoot walking on grass for 20 minutes a day can help regulate your body's electrical charge and reduce stress markers.

- **Spice up your meals:** Turmeric, ginger and cinnamon aren't just flavours, they're anti-inflammatory powerhouses.
- **Manage stress on the go:** Try box breathing (inhale for 4 seconds, hold for 4, exhale for 4, hold for 4) or step outside for 5 minutes of sunlight to reset your nervous system.
- **Eat colour, not beige:** The more colour on your plate, the more antioxidants and polyphenols you feed your body.
- **Move often:** Short bursts of activity keep blood sugar stable and improve hormone sensitivity.

Consistency beats complexity. Nail these daily and your chemistry starts to work for you, not against you.

Chapter Summary

The chapter showed how chemistry shapes regeneration from the inside out: every meal, supplement, medication, environment exposure and hormone signal influences whether your body trends towards repair or breakdown. Once you understand that chemistry is running in the background all day, you can start designing it on purpose rather than hoping it behaves.

We explored the idea of precision over volume. Supplements, powders and wellness trends create noise, while testing creates clarity. Blood markers, inflammation signals, glucose control, lipid balance, thyroid function and key nutrients give you a usable picture of what your body needs right now. This turns health into a feedback loop: measure, adjust, re-check, improve.

Hormones were positioned as master switches that influence energy, mood, sleep, recovery and body composition. You covered the big players, how they interact, and why life stages like menopause and midlife shifts require a strategy rather than willpower. The core point stayed consistent: stable chemistry makes everything easier.

Food was treated as chemical instruction, not calories. Protein, fibre, fats, polyphenols and micronutrients each push different pathways, especially inflammation and blood sugar stability. You also tackled the common traps: trend-led fixes, supplement overload and relying on guesswork instead of data.

The chapter then moved into advanced chemistry and delivery: peptides, IV therapy, and longer-horizon biotech, with a clear message that foundations come first and advanced tools work best when the internal environment is prepared.

This is where the Regen PhD Pod fits. It supports delivery and uptake by shifting the body into a receptive state and improving how inputs reach tissues. Chemistry becomes more effective when the delivery pathway is upgraded.

Core theme: test, design, repeat.

Chemistry is the controllable environment your regeneration depends on.

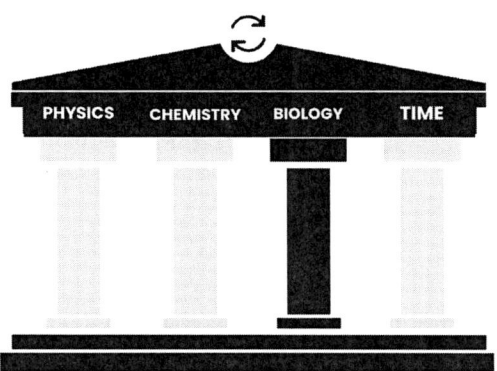

Pillar 3 - Biology: You Are Not a Machine

"We treat the body like a car. It's not. It's a forest."

"I think the tree is an element of regeneration which in itself is a concept of time."

Joseph Beuys

Biology – The Science of Human Living

Most people like the car analogy because it feels controllable. When something breaks, you replace the part and move on. That way of thinking helps when we talk about structure, load and mechanical failure.

Biology is different. Your body is not a garage project; it is a living system with roots and branches, signals and seasons, where one change reshapes something else entirely and pulling a single thread sends movement through the whole fabric.

Physics gives you force and structure, Chemistry gives you inputs and reactions now Biology is how the whole thing stays alive. It is the conversation between gut and brain, hormones and sleep, immunity shifts and repair cycles. It doesn't clock off; nor does it wait for your calendar to clear. It adapts to whatever you throw at it, until it cannot.

Think of a forest. You can see the trees but you cannot see the mycelium web under the ground, moving nutrients and messages in every direction. That is biology. It is the hidden network that lets you heal, think, sleep and move without falling apart. Ignore it and you get the slow fade: energy drops, mood swings, weight fluctuations and lingering pain. You chase symptoms in circles because you are looking at trunks, not roots.

This pillar is built from five areas
- Digestion
- Hormones
- Rhythm
- Sleep
- Nervous system

These areas do not operate as isolated units. They trade signals constantly, shaping one another's behaviour from moment to moment. The microbes in your gut produce chemicals that influence your brain. Your stress state alters the way you digest and absorb nutrients. Your sleep pattern dictates the timing and precision of hormone release. Your hormonal balance affects the speed of tissue repair. Each system adjusts to the others in real time, creating a network of responses rather than separate processes. The body can compensate for imbalance for a period, although eventually that compensation reaches a limit, and the strain becomes visible.

A quick reality check: you can't whiteknuckle your way through this, you can't out-supplement bad sleep, you can't meditate your way past iron deficiency and you can't foam roll a nervous system stuck in threat.

How this will work:
1. **Make the invisible visible.**
   Signs matter before scans: the state of your skin, stools, libido, body temperature, resting heart rate and morning stiffness. These are your early data points, then add numbers when needed. Check bloods, wearables and motion analysis not because gadgets are cool but because guessing is pointless.
2. **Reduce noise.**
   Your biology hates chaos – irregular meals, pinging phones, blue light at midnight or five coffees before lunch. Strip out noise and your systems will resync faster.
3. **Dose inputs on purpose.**
   Food, light, motion, heat, cold, breath, these are levers. The right dose at the right time changes chemistry which changes biology. We keep it simple and repeatable.
4. **Track responses, not vibes.**
   You will get a toolkit at the end of each section, short things that work when you actually do them.

A note on psychological trauma.

When a system has lived through significant stress, the body adapts by staying ready for threat. This is not a question of attitude; it is a physiological shift involving nerves, hormones and immune pathways that have learned to protect you at all times. A system that has lived in survival mode cannot be forced into calm. It requires consistent signals of safety, predictable rhythms and small, reliable experiences of success that the body can recognise. The work in this chapter will show you how those conditions can be created in a way the nervous system can trust.

A note on menopause and the midlife shift.
Midlife is not a test of character; it is physiology changing the conditions you live in. Hormonal shifts alter sleep, heat tolerance, joint comfort, tendon behaviour and body composition, even when your habits have not changed. None of this signals failure. It reflects a system that is asking for different inputs, clearer support and more precision. This phase of life deserves a framework that matches the biology rather than a narrative of blame, and the guidance in this chapter is designed with that in mind.

Why does this matter now?

People are living longer, yet many reach midlife with bodies that feel as if they are ageing faster than expected. That mismatch creates frustration, and quick fixes rarely solve it. The solution lies in understanding the pattern rather than chasing symptoms: knowing when the body needs fuel, when it needs rest, when it needs strength and when it needs recovery. Once the pattern becomes recognisable, the sense of firefighting fades, and you gain the ability to steer your system with confidence rather than reacting to every change.

What success looks like (it's boring and brilliant but no 5am club!)

This is what well-regulated biology looks like. None of it is dramatic. None of it belongs on a wellness poster. It is simply the quiet, reliable rhythm of a system that is working.

- You wake before your alarm with a clear head and a steady mood.
- Your appetite follows a pattern you can trust.
- Digestion is regular and unremarkable.
- Your cycle or midlife transition follows a predictable rhythm.
- Training sessions leave you energised rather than exhausted.
- Emotional steadiness becomes the default rather than the exception.
- Pain appears rarely, resolves quickly and has clear triggers.

The BBB Club: Biological, Boring & Brilliant

Digestion

> *"Your digestive system is not a sewer pipe.*
> *It's mission control for your health."*

If the forest analogy holds, your digestive tract is the soil. Healthy soil is teeming with life – worms, fungi, bacteria, organic matter – each one playing a role in nourishing the trees, feeding the undergrowth and keeping the whole ecosystem in balance. Strip that soil of nutrients, kill the biodiversity, or pollute it and the forest still stands for a while… until one day, it withers away.

Your **intestinal system** is exactly that kind of living soil. It's not simply a food chute where breakfast goes in, energy comes out and waste gets flushed. It is an active control centre, biochemical, neurological and immunological, that influences every other system in your body.

- **Biochemical:** Your digestive network is a chemical factory. Enzymes, acids, bile and microbial metabolites are constantly breaking food into nutrients, synthesising vitamins and producing short-chain fatty acids that travel through your bloodstream to power cells and regulate inflammation. The chemical output of your intestinal environment can directly affect

your metabolism, hormone balance and even your brain chemistry.
- **Neurological:** Through the gut-brain axis, your digestive system communicates with your central nervous system in real time. The vagus nerve acts like a phone line, carrying updates about hunger, fullness, safety, or stress. Your enteric nervous system, often called your "second brain", holds over 500 million neurons that influence mood, decision-making and reflex responses without you even being aware.
- **Immunological:** Around 70% of your immune system is housed within the intestinal wall. Specialised immune cells line this barrier, constantly sampling what comes through: food, bacteria or toxins, and deciding whether to tolerate, attack or ignore. The intestinal **immune network** is your border control, preventing harmful invaders from entering while training your body to coexist peacefully with beneficial microbes.

This three-way role means your digestive system is a hub where chemistry, nerve signalling and immune defence intersect. If the system falters in any one of these areas, the effects ripple outwards into energy, mood, recovery, resilience and long-term health.

Right now, inside you, trillions of microbes, bacteria, fungi, viruses and archaea are working. Collectively called the microbiome, they outnumber your human cells. They manufacture vitamins, help break down food your enzymes can't handle alone, regulate your immune system and send constant messages to your brain.

This is not "alternative health" territory, this is established science. Roughly 90% of your serotonin, the neurotransmitter most famous for influencing mood, is produced in the gut, not the brain. There is a two-way conversation happening between your digestive tract and your nervous system, 24 hours a day.

That means a gut problem can show up far away from your stomach. The tension headache you've been blaming on your computer screen could actually be the result of chronic constipation. Waste matter sitting too long in the bowel releases compounds that your liver and immune system have to process. This in turn can trigger inflammation and change how your blood vessels behave, setting off that dull, pounding pain behind your eyes. Fix the constipation and the "mystery" headaches disappear without touching your caffeine intake or screen time.

If your gut is in distress, the rest of you is too, even if you haven't yet noticed, or even if the symptoms are popping up somewhere you'd never think to connect.

Why the Gut Leads in Biology

When the digestive system is unstable, every other part of the body is pushed into compensation.

Hormones: Your microbiome plays a role in metabolising oestrogen, balancing cortisol output and influencing insulin sensitivity. A disrupted digestive system can trigger hormone imbalances that ripple through energy, mood and reproductive health.

Oscillation rhythms: Your intestinal microbes keep their own circadian cycles. They influence immune timing, metabolic rate and even how well you sleep.

Sleep: Digestive health and sleep form a feedback loop; poor digestive function can damage sleep quality and poor sleep disrupts gut microbial diversity.

Trauma/nervous system: The gut brain axis, via the vagus nerve and immune signalling, means stress and trauma alter digestive function and intestinal inflammation feeds back into stress response.

The Science Beneath the Surface

1. **Microbial diversity**
   A healthy microbiome is like a well-staffed city: engineers, cleaners, emergency responders, builders and administrators, each with a job that keeps the city running smoothly. Low diversity means entire departments shut down. Nutrient extraction falters, waste management slows and opportunistic "gang" microbes move into empty buildings.

Why it matters: Without enough diversity, the body becomes more vulnerable to infections, nutrient deficiencies, chronic inflammation and metabolic disorders. Studies have found that people with low microbial diversity are more likely to experience obesity, depression, autoimmune conditions and even accelerated biological ageing. It's the difference between a thriving metropolis and a run-down ghost town.

2. **Short-chain fatty acids (SCFAs)**
   When beneficial bacteria ferment dietary fibre, they produce short-chain fatty acids, notably butyrate, acetate and propionate, which act like chemical currency, paying for critical maintenance work across your body.
   - Butyrate fuels the cells lining your colon, keeping them strong and leak-proof. It also calms inflammation and even supports brain health by crossing the blood-brain barrier.
   - Acetate helps regulate appetite signals, influencing how full you feel after a meal. It also supports the

immune system's tolerance training, teaching it what are threats and what are not.
  - Propionate assists in balancing blood sugar and lowering cholesterol production in the liver.

Why it matters: SCFAs are not just "waste products" from bacteria, they are active messengers and repair agents. Without enough of them, intestinal barrier strength drops, inflammation rises and your metabolism can lose its rhythm.

3. **Intestinal permeability**
   Your intestinal lining is a single cell thick, about as delicate as tissue paper and the "tight junctions" between those cells act like doormen at an exclusive club, deciding who gets in and who stays out. Under ideal conditions, they let nutrients pass into the bloodstream while keeping toxins, pathogens and undigested food particles contained.

Stress, alcohol, certain medications, infections and poor diet can loosen these junctions, a state often called "leaky gut". When that happens, harmful substances slip into circulation. Your immune system detects them and reacts, sometimes overreacting, creating a background hum of inflammation that can affect joints, skin, brain and energy levels.

Why it matters: Chronic, low-grade inflammation from a leaky gut is now linked to a laundry list of modern conditions, from brain fog and fatigue to autoimmune flares and cardiovascular disease.

4. **Microbial circadian rhythm**
   Your microbes aren't passive passengers; they work in shifts. Certain bacterial species dominate in the morning to help break down breakfast; others clock in later to deal with lunch or dinner and some handle overnight maintenance.

Disrupt your eating times, live on shift work, or stay up late regularly and you throw their schedule off. When microbial timing goes haywire, digestion suffers, immune regulation stumbles and sleep-wake cycles get scrambled.

Why it matters: The intestinal circadian rhythm is one reason late-night snacking often leads to digestive upset, poor sleep and weight gain – your microbial workforce is literally off duty. Aligning your eating patterns with daylight hours can improve digestion, energy and even mood stability.

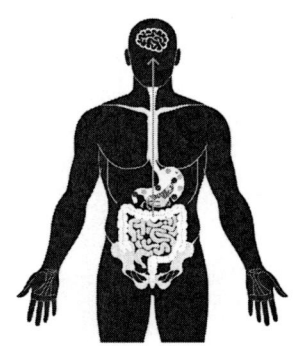

Regeneration Starts Here

How you build resilience (diversity):
Every new plant food you introduce brings a different set of fibres and polyphenols, and each of those becomes fuel for a different microbial species. Diversity grows when your diet expands, not when it stays predictable. The simplest way to build resilience is to add one new plant, herb or spice each day or each week, because each addition feeds a new branch of your microbial community. As those species grow, they provide redundancy, so if one metabolic pathway slows, another takes over, which is why athletes with broad microbial diversity recover faster and experience fewer injuries. Resilience is not something you buy, it is something you feed consistently.

How you trigger repair signals (SCFAs):
Short-chain fatty acids such as butyrate appear when microbes ferment resistant starches and soluble fibres that reach the colon intact. You create these signals by choosing foods that your enzymes cannot fully break down: cooled potatoes, lentils, oats, onions, apples and flax are reliable sources. When these foods appear regularly in your diet, microbial fermentation rises and butyrate production

increases. Butyrate supports the cells lining the colon, tightens the junctions that keep the intestinal wall sealed and down-regulates inflammatory genes. Each of these steps forms a direct signal for the body to shift from defence into repair.

How you stabilise energy control (intestinal integrity):
A sealed intestinal lining changes the way your immune system behaves. You support that lining by eating foods that increase butyrate, and by providing nutrients such as omega-3 fats and zinc that help maintain the structure of the barrier. A strong barrier prevents bacterial fragments, especially LPS (Lipopolysaccharides), from leaking into the bloodstream. When that leak is reduced, the immune system stops spending its time responding to false alarms. The result is better mitochondrial output, because mitochondria can focus on producing ATP for movement, repair and cognitive function rather than diverting resources to inflammation.

How you improve timing (circadian intestinal rhythm):
Your microbes respond to light, darkness and feeding patterns. You support their timing by eating at consistent times and aligning your largest meal with daylight. This allows microbial metabolites such as acetate and propionate to rise when your natural repair hormones, including growth hormone and melatonin, are active. Late-night grazing interrupts this rhythm and pushes microbial activity into the wrong phase, which weakens the synergy between digestion, repair and metabolic control. Consistency in mealtimes is a practical way to give the intestinal clock a stable rhythm.

When the Gut Falls Apart

Modern living is a hostile environment for your microbiome:
- Ultra-processed foods starve beneficial bacteria and feed inflammatory species.
- Antibiotics essential when needed can wipe out whole bacterial populations indiscriminately.
- Chronic stress alters blood flow to the digestive tract, slows digestion and shifts the microbiome's balance.
- Poor sleep disrupts gut microbial diversity.
- Low-fibre diets deprive bacteria of the raw material for SCFA production.
- Sedentary lifestyles slow intestinal motility and waste clearance.

Real-Life example

Sarah, 44, thought she was doing everything right. Three early-morning runs a week. A yoga class on Sundays. Protein bars in her handbag "just in case". Carbs avoided unless they were wrapped in lettuce leaves. Her friends saw her as the one with discipline.

Yet her body wasn't buying it. By mid-morning she was already bloated, her knees throbbed after every run and the familiar 3pm crash arrived like clockwork: foggy brain, short temper, a quiet urge to lie down somewhere dark. Her GP told her it was "probably stress".

Sarah came to me about her knees, thinking that running had impacted them. I asked her to track her food and symptoms for two weeks, then the picture sharpened. She was eating fewer than ten different plant foods in an average week. Most days, her "clean" protein bars were her main snack, loaded with emulsifiers, sweeteners and barely a gram of fibre. Meals were built around chicken, eggs and salad leaves – technically healthy but offering her microbiome almost nothing to work with.

We started small; the protein bars went and in their place came whole-food snacks: a handful of almonds, sliced apple with nut butter and carrot sticks with hummus. Each week she added three new plant foods: chickpeas, blueberries and pumpkin seeds. By week four, she was hitting over 30 varieties, including herbs and spices.

To address her bloating, we introduced a targeted probiotic strain, Bifidobacterium lactis HN019, shown in research to help reduce bloating, speed up bowel transit time and support the intestinal lining, this was chosen to match her symptoms and test results. We also brought in resistant starch sources like cooled potatoes and lentils. When cooked potatoes are cooled, some of their starch changes into a form your digestive enzymes can't break down. This resistant starch passes through to the large intestine, where beneficial bacteria ferment it into butyrate, the fuel that keeps the colon lining healthy, leak-proof and less inflamed. The best part? You can reheat cooled potatoes without losing the resistant starch to feed the butyrate-producing bacteria.

At first, she was sceptical but eight weeks in, her knee pain had dropped by 40%, bloating was an occasional blip rather than a daily feature and that crushing 3pm slump was gone. She even started walking after lunch, not because it was on the plan but she actually had the energy and felt lighter.

The shift went beyond symptoms. Her mood evened out, she began sleeping more deeply and her running pace improved without adding a single extra workout. All from changing what was on her plate and, more importantly, what was feeding the microscopic city inside her digestive system.

Sarah's story is proof that a "healthy" diet isn't defined by marketing labels or calorie counts, it's about diversity, balance and giving your internal ecosystem the raw materials it needs to work for you instead of against you.

Even better, she did not need any kind of medical intervention for her knees, which in the long run could have affected her whole-body regeneration.

Your Gut Talks and Your Brain Listens

Your digestive system isn't working in isolation. It's in constant conversation with your brain through what scientists call the gut brain axis.

Vagus nerve: This is the high-speed cable between your digestive tract and your brain. When the digestive tract is inflamed, the signal weakens, which can heighten anxiety, dull your mood, or leave you feeling flat.

Immune pathways: Inflammation in the intestine triggers chemical messengers (cytokines) that travel through the bloodstream and influence brain chemistry.

Hormonal signals: Your digestive system also plays a part in controlling hunger hormones like ghrelin and leptin, and stress hormones like cortisol, all of which affect mood, focus and resilience.

This is why constipation can give you a headache, why intestinal inflammation can trigger brain fog and why healing the digestive system often improves mood without a single "mindset" exercise.

Food Is More Than Fuel, It's Code for Your Microbiome

Every bite you take sends instructions to your intestinal bacteria.
- Fibre-rich plants feed the species that make short-chain fatty acids (SCFAs), lowering inflammation and supporting a healthy intestinal lining.
- Polyphenols in berries, cocoa, coffee and olive oil act as antioxidants and feed beneficial microbes.
- Refined sugar and certain fats can encourage pro-inflammatory species and crowd out the ones that protect you.

Knowing Beats Guessing

You can make big changes just by tracking how you feel after meals, but testing gives you a sharper picture:
- Food/symptom diary for spotting patterns and quick wins.
- Stool microbiome testing to see microbial diversity and SCFA potential (best interpreted with a professional).
- Blood markers like C-reactive protein for inflammation, plus checks on nutrient and thyroid status.

A practical tool for gut awareness

The Gut Tracker turns these concepts into practical, measurable behaviour. For two minutes a day you record meals, symptoms, energy, mood and sleep, and the patterns begin to surface. When this log is linked with MAI-Motion activity data, you can see how small choices influence your system, such as the way a fifteen-minute walk after lunch steadies afternoon energy or how late eating alters digestive comfort the following morning. Over time you shift from guessing to making decisions informed by your own biology. A downloadable version of this tracker will be available from the website.

I have provided some sample trackers here to give you and idea of what to look at. You can download these and more from my website.

Daily Tracker

Date	
Sleep Quality (poor / fair / good / excellent)	
Wake-up Energy (low / fair / steady / strong)	
Meals	**Comment what you have eaten and portion size**
Breakfast	
Lunch	
Dinner	
Snacks	

Symptoms	Tick/Add Notes
Bloating	
Gas	
Cramps	
Reflux (acid)	
Nausea	
Constipation	
Loose stools	
Other	

Pillar 3 - Biology: You Are Not a Machine

Energy Levels (Low, Moderate, High) Time of Day	Notes
Morning	
Noon	
Night	
Mood Check	**Notes**
(calm / steady / irritable / flat / anxious / motivated)	
Movement Activity	**Notes**
Steps	
Exercise / activity	
Bowel Movement Detail	**Entry**
Time	
Type (1 to 7)	
Ease (easy / slow / strained)	
General Notes	

Weekly Gut Summary

Category	Entry
Week Commencing	
Overall Sleep	
Overall Energy	
Main Symptoms This Week	
Foods Linked to Improvements	
Foods Linked to Discomfort	
Stress Levels	
Movement Levels	
Medicines or Supplements	
Notes on Bowel Habits	
Most Helpful Change This Week	
Focus for Next Week	
General Notes	

Pillar 3 - Biology: You Are Not a Machine

2 Minute Tracker

Date	Entry
Meals (quick notes)	
Symptoms (0 to 3)	
Energy (0 to 5)	
Mood (one word)	
Bowel Movement (type)	
Sleep Quality	
General Notes	

These trackers and more (plus all of the worksheets in this book) can be downloaded here

From Theory to Action: The 14-Day Gut Reset

Week 1 - Foundation

- **Day 1–3:** Swap processed breakfasts (cereal, bars, pastries) for oats, chia pudding, or eggs with vegetables. Aim for 2L of water daily.

- **Day 4–5:** Add one fermented food daily (yoghurt, kefir, sauerkraut, kimchi) if you tolerate it.

- **Day 6–7:** Walk 10 minutes after lunch and dinner to aid digestion; add one new vegetable this week.

Week 2 - Diversity and Timing

- **Day 8–9:** Add resistant starch sources such as cooled potatoes, lentils, or green bananas.

- **Day 10–11:** Remove alcohol and added sugar completely for two days.

- **Day 12:** Introduce two new spices or herbs.

- **Day 13–14:** Align meals with daylight hours to support your microbes' circadian rhythm.

Track your changes with my Gut Tracker or a simple notebook: note meals, symptoms, mood and sleep. By Day 14, you'll see patterns and often, results you can feel.

Gut Myths That Waste Time

Before you start, clear these from your mental hard drive:
- **"You need a detox."** Your liver and kidneys detox you 24/7. If they stop, you need an ER, not celery juice.
- **"All probiotics work the same."** Benefits are strain-specific; the wrong strain won't touch your problem.
- **"Gluten is toxic for everyone."** Only an issue in coeliac disease or non-coeliac gluten sensitivity. Whole grains benefit most people.
- **"Constipation means low fibre."** Could be low hydration, high stress, low magnesium, or thyroid dysfunction.
- **"White bread, rice and pasta are 'bad' carbs."** They're lower in fibre than wholegrain versions but they're not inherently harmful. In fact, cooling cooked white rice or potatoes increases resistant starch, which feeds beneficial bacteria. It's the dietary pattern that matters, a mix of whole grains, resistant starches and fibre-rich plants is the real win for your gut.

Common Gut Questions

Q: Should I cut carbs to heal my gut?
No, your microbiome thrives on complex carbs and fibre from fruits, vegetables, legumes and whole grains. Cutting them starves beneficial bacteria, especially those that produce short-chain fatty acids (SCFAs), which protect your gut lining and regulate inflammation. Low-carb diets can sometimes reduce bloating temporarily but in the long run they can *weaken* your gut's resilience.

Q: Can I fix my gut in a week?
You can often ease symptoms in days, for example, by removing an obvious trigger food or improving hydration. Rebuilding a diverse, resilient microbiome takes weeks to months of consistent habits. Think of it like planting a garden: you can clear the weeds fast, but it takes a season for the soil and plants to truly thrive.

Q: Are artificial sweeteners harmful?
The research is mixed. Some sweeteners (like saccharin and sucralose) can alter the microbiome in ways linked to glucose intolerance in animal studies. Others, like stevia or monk fruit, appear gentler. The safest approach is moderation,

occasional use is unlikely to cause problems for most people but relying on them daily may shift your microbial balance over time.

Q: Should I take digestive enzymes?

Only if you have a diagnosed deficiency or condition (like pancreatic insufficiency) where they're genuinely needed. For most people, simple strategies improve digestion: chew food thoroughly, eat without distractions, manage stress at meals and focus on a wide range of whole foods. These steps help your body produce and use its own enzymes efficiently.

Q: Should I do a colon cleanse?

In a word: no. Your colon doesn't need "flushing", it's self-cleaning when you're eating enough fibre, staying hydrated and moving regularly. Colon cleanses can strip away beneficial bacteria, irritate the gut lining and in rare cases cause serious complications. If you're constipated, focus on hydration, dietary fibre, movement and stress management before considering anything more invasive.

Q: Does intermittent fasting help the gut?

It can, for some people. Time-restricted eating (like 12–16 hours between your last and first meal) may give the gut lining a rest, support microbial circadian rhythms and improve blood sugar control. The benefits come from consistency and nutrient quality, not from extreme fasting windows. If fasting leaves you fatigued, anxious, or overeating later, it's not serving your gut health.

Practical Toolkit

Resistant starch booster:

Include 2–3 servings a week of cooled starchy foods such as potatoes, sweet potatoes, rice or pasta. Cook them, let them cool completely (at least 4 hours in the fridge), then eat cold (as in a salad) or reheat. Cooling changes some of the starch into *resistant starch*, which feeds beneficial gut bacteria and increases butyrate production. Butyrate is essential for keeping your gut barrier strong and reducing chronic inflammation.

Daily non-negotiables:
- Eat 5+ plant varieties
- Hydrate according to output and aim for roughly one bathroom visit per drink (6 drinks = 6 trips to the toilet) rather than chasing an arbitrary litre target
- Take 10+ minutes for mindful eating
- Walk after meals

Weekly:
- Add one new plant food
- Review gut tracker data
- Spend time outdoors

Intermediate:
- Track fibre intake (25–35g/day)
- Include resistant starch daily
- Take a break from ultra-processed foods

Advanced:
- Microbiome testing
- Gut-hormone tracking
- Timed feeding for circadian alignment

Closing Takeaway

Your gut isn't a straight tube; it's a living, reactive interface between the outside world and your cells. It's a living, talking, decision-making ecosystem. Feed it, protect it and it will keep the rest of your forest alive and thriving. Neglect it and you'll be trying to nurture your health on barren soil.

Hormones: The Timing System of Regeneration

We've already crossed paths with hormones back in Chemistry but here in Biology they take centre stage as the *master timing system* for your entire regeneration process.

Hormones tell your cells when to start repair mode, when to build muscle, when to turn down inflammation, when to store energy and when to burn it. They set the pace for your recovery after training, decide how well you sleep and even influence whether your immune system is on high alert or standing down.

The thing about hormones is they rarely change suddenly. They shift gradually, until one day you realise the rules have changed. What used to be a week to bounce back from a heavy load now takes a fortnight. Weight starts creeping on without changing your diet. Sleep gets lighter, energy flatter and mood a little more unpredictable. It's not necessarily anything you've done; it's the body adjusting its entire repair schedule.

Some of those shifts are part of life's natural seasons: menopause, andropause, the gradual changes in growth hormone, thyroid function and cortisol regulation that come with age. Others are self-inflicted, driven by chronic stress, poor sleep, overtraining, under-recovery or missing key nutrients. In both cases, the outcome is the same: repair slows and wear-and-tear gets the upper hand.

Here's the bit people miss, hormones are *responsive*. They react to your daily inputs. Light exposure, meal timing, training rhythm, how you deal with stress, even the consistency of your sleep all feed directly into your hormonal signals. Get the inputs right and your repair system speeds up. Get them wrong and you're effectively telling your body to age faster.

Basically, this section isn't about "balancing" hormones in some vague wellness sense. It's about learning how to work with your own timing system, so regeneration stays ahead of breakdown, no matter your age or stage. This is the difference between feeling like you're constantly playing catch-up and feeling like your body is one step ahead, fixing problems before they become symptoms.

Hormones & Regeneration - The Chemical Timing System

If the gut is the soil in our forest, then hormones are the seasons. They decide not just what grows but when, triggering bursts of repair, times of rest and moments of renewal. You can have fertile ground and perfect conditions but if the seasons are out of sync, growth stalls, repair slows and the whole ecosystem feels out of balance.

Hormones aren't just about mood swings or libido. They're the master schedule for regeneration, governing bone strength, muscle repair, immune resilience and even how quickly your body bounces back from stress or injury. When they're in sync, repair happens almost without effort. When they're not, it can feel like you're doing everything "right" and still getting nowhere.

You should know that hormonal harmony isn't a default setting. It's dynamic, changing by the hour, by the season and by the decade. Your regeneration potential changes right along with it.

1. Hormones as Repair Signals

Most people think of hormones in the "headline" sense: oestrogen, testosterone, cortisol and insulin. However, underneath that are dozens of others, each acting like a trigger for specific repair and regeneration programmes.

Growth hormone (GH) isn't just for bodybuilders. It spikes while you're in deep sleep, telling your body to repair muscle, reinforce bone and replace damaged cells. Miss out on deep sleep and you literally miss your nightly regeneration window.

What you can do: Prioritise a consistent bedtime window, especially the hours before midnight, when deep sleep is most easily achieved. Cool your bedroom, reduce light exposure before bed and avoid late heavy meals to maximise GH release.

Thyroid hormones are your cellular speed setting. T3 and T4 decide how quickly cells produce energy, which means they decide how fast repair work happens. Too slow and even small injuries or micro-damage from training take forever to heal.

What you can do: As noted previously, in the UK, most NHS checks will only measure TSH (thyroid-stimulating hormone). That's like checking if the manager is at their desk without asking if the workers are actually doing the job. T4 and T3 tests usually require a private panel. If you can't get these, track symptoms like cold intolerance, fatigue, slow recovery and weight changes, and bring a clear record to your GP to strengthen your case for further testing. In the meantime, support your thyroid with adequate protein, selenium (Brazil nuts, eggs, fish), iodine (seafood, seaweed) and by avoiding long-term calorie restriction.

Sex hormones such as oestrogen, progesterone and testosterone, have massive repair roles outside of reproduction. Oestrogen helps keep bones strong and arteries flexible. Progesterone is anti-inflammatory and helps you access restorative sleep. Testosterone helps maintain muscle mass, which is itself a repair asset because muscle tissue is an endocrine organ; it talks back to your hormones.

What you can do: Track symptoms like mood, libido, recovery speed and sleep quality alongside training performance. If you see persistent dips, get your levels checked and consider nutrition, training and medical options for optimisation.

Cortisol is a double-edged sword. In the right doses, it's anti-inflammatory and helps you respond to acute stress. In the wrong doses (chronically elevated), it blocks regeneration, breaks down muscle and keeps your body in a low-grade emergency state.

What you can do: Build recovery breaks into your day. Incorporate stress-buffering practices like controlled breathing, low-intensity walks, or short naps to keep cortisol from staying chronically elevated.

Your hormones don't work in isolation. They cross-talk. A cortisol spike can block testosterone production. Low progesterone can unbalance oestrogen. Poor thyroid function can flatten growth hormone output. This is why "fixing" one hormone in isolation often fails, regeneration is a team sport.

What you can do: Think systems, not single fixes. Test multiple markers together and look for patterns, rather than chasing one "hormone hack" in isolation.

2. The Regeneration Disruptors

Here's the unglamorous truth: most regeneration failures aren't because of rare hormone diseases. They're because your daily rhythms, stress loads and recovery patterns have been chipping away at your chemical timing for years.

Most of these we have already discussed but you can see them here together giving you the full picture.

Chronic stress keeps cortisol high, which not only blocks repair but also blunts the sensitivity of your cells to other hormones. It's like shouting so loudly that no one else in the room can get a word in.

What you can do: Build in "off switches" during the day, short walks without your phone, breathwork, or even 5–10 minutes of eyes-closed stillness. The goal isn't to eliminate stress but to give your system daily dips so cortisol can reset.

Circadian disruption such as late nights, screen light at midnight and erratic wake times, confuses your hormonal clock. Hormones run on patterns, not random bursts. Melatonin needs darkness, cortisol needs a morning spike and an evening dip and growth hormone needs deep, early sleep. Break the timing and even if your hormone levels look "normal" on a blood test, they're firing at the wrong times.

What you can do: Anchor your wake time first (even on weekends), limit blue light exposure 1-2 hours before bed and aim to get outside within 30 minutes of waking to lock in your morning cortisol rhythm.

Nutrient gaps blunt hormone production. Your body can't make steroid hormones without cholesterol. You need zinc for testosterone, iodine for thyroid hormones and magnesium for over 300 enzyme reactions, many of which control hormone receptors.

What you can do: Eat a varied diet with whole-food sources of these nutrients: shellfish, eggs, oily fish, nuts, seeds and dairy if tolerated. If you're plant-based, you may need targeted supplementation for zinc, iodine and B12.

Overtraining is a sneaky one. Too much intensity without enough recovery drives cortisol up and testosterone down. You don't get fitter, you get hormonally flatlined.

What you can do: Swap some high-intensity sessions for lower-intensity, restorative training (mobility work, zone 2 cardio, yoga). Track resting heart rate and energy levels, if both are climbing in the wrong direction, recovery is overdue.

3. Life-Stage Shifts, Menopause, Andropause and Drift

In the Chemistry pillar we broke down the symptoms and the politics of menopause and andropause. Here, we're looking purely at the regeneration impact.

Menopause means a significant drop in oestrogen and progesterone. This means reduced bone density; lower collagen production for joints and skin; and less anti-inflammatory buffering. It's why joint pain, slower muscle recovery and skin changes often accelerate after menopause. Without a strategy, your repair capacity takes a hit.

What you can do: Strength training is your best bone-building tool. Combine that with adequate protein (at least 1.2–1.6g per kg bodyweight) and don't skip healthy fats – they're raw material for hormone production. Discuss options like HRT with a qualified practitioner if symptoms or recovery are impacting your life.

Andropause in men, the gradual decline in testosterone, shifts the balance towards muscle loss, increased fat storage and slower recovery from training or injury.

What you can do: Resistance training at least 2–3 times per week, with compound lifts, is proven to boost testosterone. Prioritise sleep, manage stress and keep body fat in a healthy range; excess fat tissue can convert testosterone into oestrogen.

Age-related drift happens to everyone. Growth hormone peaks in your teens, then slowly declines. Melatonin production falls, making sleep shallower. DHEA, a hormone linked to resilience and anti-ageing processes, also declines. The good news is that decline is not collapse. Lifestyle inputs can maintain or even improve the function of your hormonal network, even if absolute levels dip.

What you can do: Protect your sleep window, especially the first half of the night when growth hormone peaks. Support melatonin by getting bright morning light and minimising blue light exposure at night. For DHEA, consistent exercise, stress management and a nutrient-dense diet are your foundations; supplementation should only follow proper testing.

The Regeneration Mindset

Your hormones aren't just chemical messengers, they're the switches that decide whether your body is in "build" mode or "breakdown" mode. You can't fully control them, but you can influence them every single day.

The mistake is thinking you have to "fix" everything at once. The smarter play is to identify the biggest regeneration blocker in your life: poor sleep timing, chronic stress, nutrient gaps, no strength work and fix that first. Hormones work in networks, so improving one part of the system often lifts the whole thing.

And if there's one takeaway here, it's this: Regeneration is hormonal. You can't separate the chemistry from the biology, they are the same story told in two different languages, one in electrical signals, the other in chemical ones. When they're speaking in sync, your body knows exactly how to heal.

Hormone Repair Readiness Check

How to do it:
For each habit, tick **Yes** if you do it consistently, **No** if you don't. Each **Yes** = 1 point. Total your points at the end.

Daily Habit	Yes	No
1. I get at least 10 minutes of daylight in the morning within an hour of waking.	☐	☐
2. I sleep 7–9 hours most nights and wake without an alarm at least once a week.	☐	☐
3. I strength train at least twice a week.	☐	☐
4. I do steady-state cardio or brisk walking 3+ times a week.	☐	☐
5. I eat a palm-sized portion of protein with each main meal.	☐	☐
6. I include healthy fats daily (nuts, oily fish, olive oil, avocado).	☐	☐
7. I have at least one stress-reducing habit (breathing exercises, meditation, social time).	☐	☐
8. I avoid bright screens 60–90 mins before bed.	☐	☐
9. I keep alcohol to 3 drinks or fewer per week.	☐	☐
10. I have one full recovery day each week (light activity only).	☐	☐

Menopause / Andropause Modifier

If you're in perimenopause, post-menopause, or andropause:
- Double your **YES** score for these habits:
  - Protein first at every meal
  - Strength training twice a week
  - Morning light exposure
  - Evening wind-down (dim lights, screen-free)
  - Stress breaks during the day

Why? Your baseline hormone production is lower, so the "signal" from these actions is worth more.

Your Score:
8–10 → Your hormonal repair network is likely in good working order. Keep doing what's working and fine-tune with seasonal/life stage changes.

5–7 → Some gaps in your daily rhythms could be slowing repair. Pick 1 to 2 habits to improve over the next month.

0–4 → Your hormone timing and signals are likely under strain. Start with the basics: sleep, light, protein and movement before adding advanced strategies.

Action Checklist - Based on Your Score

If You Scored Low (0–4)
- Prioritise sleep window (asleep before 11pm) for growth hormone release.
- Get outside early every day to reset your circadian rhythm.

- Add one palm-sized protein serving to your smallest meal.
- Aim for at least 30–40 minutes of gentle movement daily, broken into whatever chunks work for you - this could be two short walks, stretching, light cycling or mobility work.

If You Scored Medium (5–7)
- Layer in resistance training if not already doing it.
- Replace one screen-heavy evening with a wind-down ritual.
- Add magnesium-rich foods (leafy greens, nuts) to support hormone function.
- Do a weekly check to track improvements.

If You Scored High (8–10)
- Maintain your rhythm but rotate training to keep hormone signals fresh.
- Add small seasonal tweaks (more daylight in summer mornings, earlier nights in winter).
- Consider advanced tracking (cycle tracking, testosterone/DHEA checks).
- Keep stress modulation consistent to prevent cortisol creep.

Rhythms - Your Body's Timekeepers

Your body does not run on motivation or willpower; it runs on timing. Beneath everything you do, from thinking to digesting to repairing, there are internal clocks that set the pace. Some run every 24 hours, some run in 90-minute waves, some stretch over weeks or seasons. These oscillation rhythms are the quiet metronomes of your biology, deciding when you release hormones, when you repair tissues, when you digest food, when you sleep and when you can actually perform.

You can eat well, train well and manage stress, but if your clocks are drifting, your internal teams arrive at the wrong time with the wrong tools. Repair slows, inflammation rises and you feel like you are working twice as hard for half the result. Rhythm is not a "nice to have". It is the foundation that determines whether your body is running efficiently or wasting energy trying to compensate.

Let's look at the rhythms that matter most: circadian, ultradian, infradian and seasonal, and show you how to align them so your body can regenerate on schedule instead of fighting itself.

Circadian Rhythm - The 24-Hour Master Clock

The circadian rhythm is your 24-hour master clock – the metronome that sets the timing for almost everything. At its centre is a small cluster of neurons in the suprachiasmatic nucleus, sitting just behind your eyes, reading light like a daily instruction manual. When this clock is anchored, every other system knows when to start its shift, when to slow down and when to repair.

How it works when aligned

Morning light signals the start of the day. Cortisol rises on cue, so you begin the morning with some energy in the tank, your digestion activates and insulin sensitivity improves. By midday, your body temperature peaks, coordination sharpens and physical performance hits its natural stride. As evening arrives and light fades, melatonin increases, your temperature drops, and your body begins its descent into repair mode. Deep sleep early in the night delivers pulses of growth hormone, collagen synthesis and immune clean-up.

What disrupts it

Late-night screens delay melatonin., erratic wake times flatten your cortisol rise and eating late forces the gut and liver into night-time work when they should be repairing. Add inconsistent light exposure, and the whole system drifts into internal jet lag.

Practical ways to anchor it

1. **Light first thing.** Within an hour of waking, get outside for 5–10 minutes. Cloudy or sunny, morning light is the signal your brain trusts.
2. **Dim the evening.** Lower lights 1–2 hours before bed. Keep screens out of the bedroom or use warm filters if you must.
3. **Wake at the same time.** Your wake time is the anchor. Even after a late night, stick to it.
4. **Kitchen curfew.** Leave 2–3 hours between your last meal and sleep.
5. **Caffeine cut-off.** Try to avoid it after 2pm. It lingers in the body for a long time and blocks the signals that help you feel ready for sleep.
6. **Cool the room.** 16–18C supports the natural temperature drop that signals deep sleep.

When circadian rhythm is in sync, your biology runs on rails. When it drifts, every system works harder than it needs to.

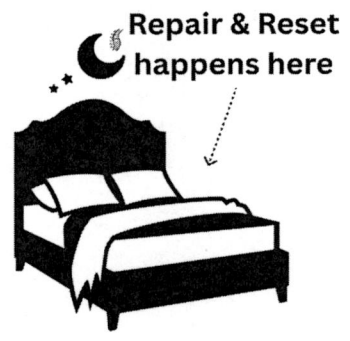

Ultradian Rhythms - The 90 to 120 Minute Waves

Circadian rhythm sets the structure of your day, but inside that structure your body runs shorter cycles called ultradian rhythms. These are waves of energy, focus and fatigue that rise and fall every 90 to 120 minutes. You have felt this pattern a thousand times. You start sharp, hit flow, then an hour or two later the edges blur. You reread the same sentence, reach for coffee or feel yourself drifting. This is your biology asking for a reset.

How ultradian rhythms work

Your brain uses these 90-minute cycles to manage resources. During the high phase, attention is strong, creativity is flexible and the nervous system is steady. As the cycle draws to a close, the brain starts signalling for a break. Ignore those cues and the system compensates by pushing stress chemistry forward, which works for a moment but costs you later.

What happens when you push through

To make sense of it, think of the acronym BURN:
- **B**oosted stress hormones – cortisol and adrenaline rise to force output.
- **U**nderpowered focus and creativity – flexibility declines, errors increase.
- **R**eserves drained – recovery systems get sidelined for longer.
- **N**ear burnout – immunity weakens, repair slows and the smallest stress hits harder.

This is one of the reasons people feel they "crash" mid-afternoon or struggle to maintain clarity late in the day.

How to work with it
1. **Block your work.** Aim for 90 minutes of deep focus, then stop. Do not wait until you are empty.
2. **Take mini-reset breaks.** Five to ten minutes is enough. Stand, stretch, breathe, get daylight, sip water. These small interruptions reset brain chemistry for the next wave.
3. **Watch your cues.** Yawning, irritability, zoning out or rereading the same line are the signals that the cycle is closing.
4. **Train to the rhythm.** Athletic performance also peaks in waves. Alternate intensity with shorter recovery drills.

Your brain is not a machine that delivers constant output, it is a wave-based system and when you work with those waves, you get more done with less strain.

Infradian Rhythms - The Long Game

Not every rhythm runs daily. Some stretch across weeks or even months, quietly shaping energy, recovery and how resilient you feel. As we've already touched on in other parts of the book, hormonal rhythms shift over time and those changes influence everything from sleep to focus to repair. Alongside these longer hormonal patterns, your body also runs on seasonal rhythms, and these become more noticeable with age.

Winter often brings lower energy, slower recovery and a heavier immune demand. Short daylight hours flatten circadian cues, joints stiffen more easily and the body naturally asks for earlier rest. Summer tends to lift energy and recovery but can also disrupt sleep with heat, longer evenings and later natural alertness.

Working with the seasons makes regeneration smoother:
- Winter responds well to vitamin D, warming foods, earlier nights and gentler training.
- Summer benefits from blackout blinds, cooler rooms, lighter meals and better hydration.
- Midday daylight helps stabilise mood and sleep in any season.

Seasonal rhythms are the longer arc of your biology. When you honour them, your energy rises and falls in a way that feels natural rather than unpredictable.

Why This Matters for Regeneration

When your internal clocks work together, repair becomes effortless. Cortisol rises on cue, melatonin triggers deep rest, growth hormone pulses overnight and your organs perform their tasks at the right time. Energy stays steady, inflammation stays low and your immune system quietly handles problems before you notice them.

When clocks drift, everything becomes harder. Hormones release at the wrong moments, digestive repair is delayed, sleep fragments, inflammation lingers, mornings feel sluggish and recovery shrinks.

The solution is alignment - the body regenerates when timing is intact.

Regeneration Rhythm Tracker

Measure. Adjust. Regenerate.

Step 1: Track Your Rhythms (1–2 weeks)

Fill in daily/weekly logs to spot where your body's clocks are drifting.

Daily Tracker

Wake time: _____

Bedtime: _____

Last meal time: _____

Screens off (time): _____

Energy peak(s): _____

Energy dip(s): _____

Reset taken? Y/N

Sleep quality (1–5): _____

Pillar 3 - Biology: You Are Not a Machine

Weekly Tracker

Average sleep/wake variance: _____

Average time between last meal & sleep: _____

Number of resets taken during workdays: _____

Seasonal energy rating (1–5): _____

Recovery markers (grip strength/HRV/resting HR): _____

Step 2: Interpret the Data

Look for patterns:
Sleep/wake times vary >90 mins → circadian misalignment

No clear 90-min dips/peaks → ignoring ultradian waves

Evening meals <2 hrs before bed → gut & liver repair delayed

Winter fatigue or summer sleep disruption → seasonal rhythms at play

Recovery markers trending down → pushing without repair

Step 3: Correct & Realign

Match what you tracked with practical fixes:

Circadian drift → lock wake time, use morning light, dim evening light

Flat ultradian waves → schedule 90-min focus blocks + 5–10 min resets

Late eating → move last meal earlier by 15 mins every few days until you hit 2–3 hrs pre-bed

Seasonal issues →
Winter: add vitamin D, earlier nights, heavier foods, slower training

Summer: blackout blinds, cool-down ritual, lighter meals

Recovery lagging → pull back on intensity, increase protein, prioritise deep sleep anchors

Step 4: Re-test

At the end of 2–4 weeks, repeat the **weekly tracker**.

Has sleep/wake variance narrowed?

Are energy waves clearer?

Has recovery (grip strength, HRV, mood) improved?
If yes → you're regenerating in sync.

If no → refine again (one variable at a time).

Stillness - Sleep as Regeneration

As the seasons shift, every forest knows when to rest. Winter slows the sap, quiets the canopy and pulls energy inwards so that growth can return stronger in spring. In the same way, sleep is our stillness, the time when energy is drawn inside, repair takes priority and your biology restores its reserves.

This is when growth hormone pulses, tissues knit back together, memory consolidates and inflammation calms down. You can eat the best food, train smart and manage stress but without deep, regular sleep, repair stalls.

Why does this matter?

Sleep is not passive downtime; it's active biological work. Every night, your body runs a tight schedule of repair jobs, hormone regulation and cognitive resets. Miss them and your health and performance slip.

- **Growth hormone release** peaks in early deep sleep. No deep sleep = no structural repair.
- **Immune clean-up** happens at night: white blood cells hunt, destroy and reset. Think of it as your body's janitorial crew.

- **Cognitive reset**: memories are filed, emotions are processed and the brain detoxifies waste proteins like beta-amyloid.
- **Hormone balance**: poor sleep drives cortisol up, testosterone/oestrogen down and wrecks insulin sensitivity, leaving you inflamed and energy-poor.

If you want regeneration, this is the non-negotiable foundation.

The Stages of Sleep And Why They Matter

Sleep functions like a team of specialists working in shifts. Each stage focuses on a different job, from memory consolidation to muscle repair. The cycle repeats every ninety minutes, and if one shift is cut short, the next team has to work harder to keep you functioning.

Stage 1 - Light Sleep (The Doorway)
This is the moment between consciousness and sleep. You're hovering, muscles relaxing, heart rate dropping, brainwaves starting to shift gears. It's quick but essential, the entry ticket. Think of it as the bouncer at the club, if you don't get past him, you're not getting inside where the real action happens.

Stage 2 - Deeper Light Sleep (The Filing Clerk)
The brain begins its basic organisational work at this stage. Short-term memories are sorted, body temperature lowers and the nervous system moves into a steadier, lower-energy state. It is not glamorous, but it is essential. Missing this stage leaves your system carrying unfinished tasks into the next day, and the result is a brain that feels overloaded before you even start.

Stage 3 - Deep (Slow-Wave) Sleep (The Restoration Phase)

This is the stage where the body does its heaviest work. Growth hormone rises, repairing the structures that carry you through the day, and the immune system uses the darkness to restore order and stability. It forms the backbone of physical regeneration. When this phase is compromised, the body begins to carry forward work it was meant to complete overnight, which gradually erodes resilience.

REM Sleep (The Mad Genius)

Your brain goes full technicolour here. Dreaming, creativity, emotional reset, memory consolidation; this is where you make sense of the day and prep for tomorrow. Without enough REM, you're less resilient, more irritable and about as creative as a damp sponge.

Each night, your body runs a cycle between **body-first repair (deep sleep)** and **brain-first repair (REM)**. Skip either one and you're trying to live at half power. Stack enough bad nights and you're basically reverse-engineering burnout.

The Environment of Sleep - Engineering the Night

Your bedroom is the environment that governs how your body enters recovery each night. Long before we understood sleep scientifically, people were adjusting their surroundings to rest well, and much of that older wisdom remains useful.

1. **Darkness**
   - The ancients knew light was a disruptor. Romans used heavy drapes, Egyptians slept in windowless stone

rooms and the Japanese perfected paper screens to control light.
- Darkness lets melatonin do its job. Even a streetlamp sneaking in through the curtains can flatten the signal. Monks in medieval monasteries slept in pitch-black cells, then rose for midnight prayers. It broke their sleep into segments but because the first stretch was in complete darkness, melatonin still had time to peak and drive deep rest.

2. **Temperature**
   - Cold nights, warm bodies. Ancient Greeks slept naked under wool blankets. In Scandinavia, children were put down for naps outside in the icy air, prams lined with blankets. The belief was simple: cold air makes for stronger, deeper sleep. Modern sleep research agrees.
   - The "hot bath before bed" trick? The Japanese ofuro (soaking baths) and Roman thermae already had this nailed centuries ago. They didn't know the word "thermoregulation", but they understood that warming the skin prepped the body for a cooler, deeper sleep.

3. **Sound**
   - Not everyone had silence. Desert cultures leaned on the sound of wind and shifting sand, while in Asia, monks engineered "soundscapes" with gongs, flutes and chants designed to drop the brain into slower rhythms.
   - Indigenous tribes often used drums or low hums as sleep rituals: vibrational white noise before white noise machines existed. Today, we call them binaural beats, but the principle hasn't changed: rhythm slows biology.

4. **Scent**
    - **Lavender** has a long history in sleep rituals: Romans stuffed pillows with it and Medieval Europeans stuffed lavender bundles into pillows to ward off restless spirits and help with sleep. Apothecaries sold it as a nerve tonic. Victorians used lavender sachets in bedding and wardrobes as it was thought to calm hysteria (a very Victorian diagnosis) and steady the nerves. And the real bonus – you can grow it so easily in your garden or window box and harvest it for free!
    - Egyptians burned **chamomile** in rituals and brewed it into calming teas. In Medieval Europe it became a staple of monastic gardens (the "physic gardens" tended by monks), used to ease insomnia, melancholy and digestive upset. It was also strewn on floors in gatherings, because when crushed it released a sweet apple-like scent thought to keep spirits high. In traditional German medicine, chamomile is known as "alles zutraut" (capable of anything), a cure-all. Germans have long used it as their go-to sleep tea. And in Ayurveda, chamomile is considered cooling and soothing, balancing "pitta" (the fire element) and used for calming restless minds at night.
    - **Frankincense**, traded like gold in ancient Arabia, was prized because burning it in temples made people calmer, slower, more meditative. Science now shows its compounds interact with the nervous system.
    - In Ayurveda, **sandalwood** paste was rubbed on the temples to "cool the mind". In Chinese medicine, mugwort smoke was used to relax muscles and "guide dreams".

- Whether or not a lab has caught up, these rituals survived because they worked, people felt calmer, slept deeper and woke clearer.

5. **Tactile Inputs**

    Sleep is physical, it's not just the brain switching off, it's the body recognising, *"I'm safe here, I can let go."* Across cultures, touch, weight and texture have been central to triggering that state.

    - **Weighted blankets** may be trending now but the idea behind them is ancient. Swaddling simply means wrapping a newborn securely, so the body feels held. Indigenous American tribes used this for safety and for the calming effect it had on infants, and the practice appears across cultures in different forms. UK maternity wards still teach swaddling because the pressure reduces startle reflexes and helps newborns settle into deeper sleep. These early patterns often carry into adulthood. People who were swaddled as infants commonly prefer bedding that feels anchored or tucked in, and many find weighted blankets naturally soothing. The physiology is the same at every age. Steady pressure signals safety to the nervous system, lowers arousal and increases the likelihood of deeper sleep. Modern sleep specialists call this "deep pressure stimulation", but it is simply a refined version of a principle humans have used for generations.
    - **Posture** - The ancient Egyptians believed posture mattered for sleep and carved headrests out of wood or stone. By modern standards they look uncomfortable, but the principle was the same as a good memory foam

pillow today: support the neck, open the airway and keep energy flow aligned. They weren't wrong; your head and neck position heavily influence the depth of your rest.
- **Natural Fibres** - Before polyester, every bed was "organic". Wool, cotton, linen, hemp – all natural fibres that breathe and regulate heat. People didn't wake drenched in sweat, because their bedding worked with them, not against them. Now, sleep scientists are circling back, showing that breathable fabrics improve temperature control, which in turn deepens sleep. Now, let's not ignore it: organic cotton, linen, or wool bedding doesn't come cheap. You can walk into a high-street shop and pick up a polyester duvet set for the price of a takeaway curry. Natural fibres – that's more like a decent weekend away. So yes, it's an investment but one that pays dividends every single night. Think of it less like "bedding" and more like buying better sleep. We'll happily spend on phones, cars, or wine without blinking but a third of your life is spent in bed. If your bedding helps you sink deeper, repair faster and wake clearer, it isn't a luxury. It's equipment for regeneration, and if the price tag really stings, start small. A single organic cotton pillowcase costs less than a full set but still gives your skin and sleep environment that breathable, natural upgrade. One swap at a time still counts.

Your body is wired to respond to physical cues: texture, pressure and alignment. These small, ancient details can turn a restless night into real regeneration.

Rituals - The Pre-Sleep Wind-Down

Regeneration thrives on rhythm. What you do in the 1–2 hours before bed sets the tone for everything that follows. Most of us treat sleep as a switch: lights off, head down and expect the body to comply. In reality, it's more like landing a plane. You need a descent pattern, not a crash landing.

1. **Light Rituals**
    - **Dim to signal dusk.** Your eyes aren't just windows; they're sensors that set your body clock. Blue light from LEDs and screens tells the brain it's noon in July, even if it's 11pm in December. No surprise melatonin doesn't show up to work.
    - **Workarounds.** If screens are non-negotiable, tech can save you from tech. Blue-light filters on phones, or amber glasses, cut the "daylight signal" enough to let your body believe it's night. Think of them as giving your hormones the memo: "shift's nearly over".

2. **Breathing and Relaxation**
    - **Nervous system brakes.** Breathing isn't just oxygen exchange; it's a remote control for your nervous system. Slow, deliberate patterns, like 4-7-8 breathing (inhale for 4, hold for 7, exhale for 8), press on the vagus nerve, telling cortisol to simmer down.
    - **Movement cues.** Gentle stretching or yin yoga can nudge muscles into rest mode. It's like closing tabs on your laptop – joints reset, muscles loosen and your body doesn't wake you at 2am because it still thinks you're stuck at your desk.

3. **Mental Unloading**
   - **Paper is therapy.** The brain hates unfinished business. Jotting down tomorrow's to-do list or today's worries tricks your prefrontal cortex into standing down. That way, your 3am self doesn't bolt awake thinking about whether you replied to that email.
   - **Reading as sedation.** Paper books (not doomscrolling) shift the mind away from input overload, bonus: if the book's boring enough, it doubles as a sedative.

4. **Ancient Practices**
   - **Ayurveda's nightcap.** Warm milk with nutmeg has been prescribed for centuries to cool fiery energy and soothe the mind. Today we might swap it for oat milk, but the principle stands: warmth plus spice equals calm.
   - **Chinese organ clocks.** Traditional Chinese Medicine teaches that each organ has a time window. The liver's 1–3am "detox shift" is legendary. Whether you buy the literal interpretation or not, the lesson is sound: get to bed *before* midnight so the body has the energy to repair, not just stay awake.
   - **Sound as sedation.** Indigenous traditions leaned on rhythm, drums, chants and rain sticks, to ease people into altered states. The modern version is sound baths, Tibetan singing bowls and binaural beats. Different costume, same function: cue the nervous system to stand down.

5. **Gratitude and Mindset**
   - Ending the day with gratitude shifts the nervous system out of stress mode. Instead of rehearsing

tomorrow's worries, you anchor into today's wins, no matter how small.
- Ancient Stoics did this with evening reflections, asking themselves, *"What did I do well today? What can I improve?"* Monks kept journals of thanks. Indigenous traditions often gave thanks to the land, the ancestors or the elements before sleep.
- Today, it can be as simple as jotting three things you're thankful for: a good meal, a laugh and a kind word. That tiny practice lowers cortisol, boosts serotonin and sets the stage for deeper rest.

Nutrition and Sleep - Feeding the Night

Food doesn't just fuel you; it *signals* to your body what time of day it is. Eat the wrong thing or eat it too late and your body clock gets scrambled. Eat the right things and you're essentially programming your system for deeper rest.

1. **Timing Matters**
   - Stop eating 2–3 hours before bed. Digestion is energy-intensive and your body can't fully repair cells and tissues while it's still busy breaking down a heavy curry or pizza.
   - Big late-night meals suppress growth hormone, one of the key drivers of cellular repair.
   - Ancient Greeks and Romans often practised "early dining", with lighter evening meals, believing that heaviness in the gut clouded the mind and spirit. Modern sleep labs back this as late-night eating shortens deep rest windows.

2. **What Helps**
   - **Magnesium**: Known as the "relaxation mineral", it soothes muscles and quiets the nervous system. Ancient Egyptians used magnesium-rich Epsom salt baths for healing. Today, leafy greens, nuts and pumpkin seeds are your allies.
   - **Tryptophan**: Found in turkey, oats, bananas and seeds, this amino acid is the raw material for serotonin and melatonin. Medieval herbalists often prescribed warm oat gruel or milk with honey at night – both naturally boost tryptophan intake.
   - **Chamomile and Passionflower**: Chamomile tea was used in ancient Egypt for calming fevers and soothing spirits. Passionflower, native to the Americas, was brewed by indigenous tribes to ease restlessness. Today, both are clinically shown to reduce sleep latency (time to fall asleep).
   - **Glycine**: Abundant in collagen-rich foods like bone broth and gelatine, glycine lowers core body temperature, a key trigger for deep sleep. Traditional Chinese Medicine often paired broth-based evening soups with herbs for exactly this reason.

3. **What Hurts**
   - **Caffeine**: With a half-life of 6–8 hours, your afternoon coffee is still active at midnight. Ancient Arabian physicians actually warned against overuse of coffee after dark when it first arrived from Ethiopia.
   - **Alcohol**: Although wine has been a sleep aid since Roman times, the reality is it only sedates, not restores. Modern science confirms what monks complained of centuries ago: night drinking causes restless, broken sleep.

- **Sugar**: Sweet treats before bed spike blood sugar and trigger rebound crashes at 3am, leading to sudden wakefulness. Ayurvedic texts warned against "heavy sweets" at night for the same reason: they disturb digestive fire and unbalance energy.

Closing - Sleep as the Master Regenerator

You can stack supplements, track every biomarker and chase the latest wellness gadgets but without sleep, regeneration remains theory. Sleep is not downtime, it's repair, hormone and immune time.

When you honour it, your body doesn't just recover from today, it lays the groundwork for tomorrow. Every system, every rhythm, every practice in this book is amplified or undermined by the quality of your sleep.

Sleep is the foundation of regeneration. Protect it, prioritise it, respect it. Everything else builds from here.

The Nervous System

The Signal Pathways of the Forest

In our forest analogy, your nervous system is the network of roots, mycelium threads and hidden channels that keep everything communicating. It's the forest's electrical grid and postal service rolled into one, sending urgent alerts, daily updates and subtle suggestions from one end of the woodland to the other.

If one tree is stressed, perhaps a pest has started eating its leaves, it sends chemical signals through the roots and mycelium to its neighbours. In a healthy forest, these signals are quick, clear and proportional to the situation. They respond by producing protective compounds before the threat even reaches them. In your body, your nervous system does exactly this: sensing, anticipating and adjusting before you consciously realise anything has changed. You don't think, my balance is slipping, I'd better shift my weight, you just adjust, instantly.

Now picture a forest that's been struck by storms, fire, or years of slow neglect. Some pathways get damaged and start sending false alarms, like a tree constantly screaming "fire!"

even though the weather is calm. Other pathways go silent, leaving patches of the forest isolated and vulnerable. That's what happens when trauma or chronic stress reshapes your nervous system.

The damage isn't always obvious. You might still be standing tall like a healthy tree but underneath the soil, the roots are strained. In human terms, that could mean your muscles stay tense even when you're safe, your digestion slows without you noticing, or your heart rate spikes at small provocations.

Most of this is handled by your autonomic nervous system, the part that keeps your heart beating, lungs inflating, hormones releasing and digestion ticking over without asking your permission. It has two main settings: the accelerator (*fight-or-flight*), which mobilises you to respond to danger and the brake (*rest-and-digest*), which restores and repairs you afterwards. Both are essential, you can't thrive without being able to speed up *and* slow down. But trauma, chronic stress and certain illnesses can trap you in one setting for too long. Stuck in overdrive, you burn through resources. Stuck in shutdown, you struggle to muster energy at all. Either way, regeneration slows.

Trauma leaves its mark everywhere in this network. In your brain, it can shrink the hippocampus (memory and learning), over-activate the amygdala (threat detection) and weaken the prefrontal cortex (planning and decision-making). In your hormone system, it can keep cortisol and adrenaline high for months or years. In your immune system, it can push inflammation into a permanent simmer and in your body, it can set in tension patterns, alter your breathing and disrupt digestion.

Pillar 3 - Biology: You Are Not a Machine

Here's the good news, and it's the reason this part of the biology chapter matters so much. Just as a damaged forest can recover when the soil is restored and the roots reconnect, your nervous system can regenerate. Neuroplasticity is biology, your brain and body genuinely can rewire when they receive the right cues. The task is giving those cues consistently, in an environment that signals safety rather than threat.

By the end of this section, you'll know what is happening beneath the surface when your nervous system becomes overwhelmed, why the effects show up everywhere from your digestion to your mood and what you can start doing today to help it rebalance, repair and return to a state that actually supports you instead of fighting against you.

The Autonomic Nervous System - The Wiring You Don't Control

Your nervous system is the control network that runs your whole body. It's the operating system beneath the surface. You don't think about raising your heart rate, slowing digestion or tightening muscles before a deadline. Your autonomic nervous system (ANS) handles that for you, constantly adjusting your internal settings based on what it thinks is happening around you.

The ANS has two main modes:
- Sympathetic nervous system (SNS): your accelerator, preparing you to act.
- Parasympathetic nervous system (PNS): your brake, restoring and repairing.

Both matter. Trouble starts when life, illness or stress trap you in one mode for too long. Too much accelerator and you live in constant alert. Too much brake and you struggle to get moving. Either state slows regeneration.

Pillar 3 - Biology: You Are Not a Machine

Beyond Fight or Flight – The Survival Programmes

Most people know fight or flight, but your nervous system actually has four main survival responses. None of them are character flaws. They are biological programmes built for protection.

1. Fight
The system powers up to confront a challenge. Useful in danger but draining when switched on all day. Headaches, tension and digestive issues often trace back to living in this mode for too long.

2. Flight
The body prepares to escape. Your heart races, your senses sharpen. Helpful when you need to get to safety. Unhelpful when everyday stressors trigger the same pattern and avoidance becomes your norm.

3. Freeze
When neither fight nor escape feels possible, the system hits pause. You may feel stuck, disconnected or unable to start tasks, it's not laziness, rather the body protecting you until it senses safety again.

4. Fawn
Some people cope with stress by appeasing or over-accommodating. It's an old survival strategy designed to keep the peace, but it is exhausting when it becomes automatic.

Understanding these modes helps you recognise what your body is doing and why certain "mystery symptoms" appear even when life looks calm on the surface.

The Vagus Nerve – Your Recovery Line

You don't need to memorise anatomy. Just remember this: your vagus nerve is the main communication line between brain and body. When it works well, you recover faster, inflammation stays lower and digestion, sleep and mood stabilise. When it's sluggish, everything becomes harder.

High vagal tone = flexible, responsive, resilient.
Low vagal tone = wired, tired and slow to repair.

The term 'vagal tone' is misleading. There's no noise involved; it's simply your nervous system's recovery speed, how quickly it can settle after being pushed. You can train it with simple cues the body recognises as safety.

Daily habits that strengthen this recovery line:
- Slow, deep breathing with long exhales
- Gentle movement like walking or stretching
- Cold splash or brief cold exposure
- Humming, singing or anything that vibrates the throat
- Warmth, sunlight, and positive social connection

These are not hacks; they are biological signals telling the system it is safe enough to shift into repair mode.

Why This Matters for Regeneration

When the nervous system is overwhelmed, every other area of biology is forced into crisis management. Digestion slows, hormones misfire, sleep fragments and inflammation rises.

When the system feels safe and responsive again, those processes fall back into rhythm and recovery accelerates.

The goal isn't to stop stress.

It's to give your body the cues it needs to switch out of survival mode and into repair more often.

Smiling, Laughter and Nervous System Recovery

One of the simplest ways to influence the nervous system is through facial expression and breath. Smiling and laughter are not just responses to feeling safe; they are physical actions that help *create* safety in the body.

When you smile or laugh, facial muscles send signals through the nervous system that shift the body away from threat and towards regulation. This activates the parasympathetic nervous system, the state in which repair, digestion and recovery can occur. Stress chemistry begins to soften and the body moves out of constant alert.

Laughter deepens this effect. It lowers cortisol, increases endorphins and supports the release of dopamine and serotonin, chemicals involved in pain relief, mood balance and emotional resilience. Breathing becomes fuller and more rhythmic, circulation improves and muscle tension that has been held unconsciously begins to release.

From a biological perspective, laughter improves oxygen delivery, gently stimulates the diaphragm and supports lymphatic flow, all of which contribute to immune health and reduced inflammation. It also improves heart rate variability, a key marker of nervous system flexibility and recovery capacity.

Trauma tightens the system. It narrows breathing, stiffens posture and keeps the body braced for what might happen next. Smiling and laughter introduce the opposite signal. They widen the system, soften protective tension and remind the nervous system that it can stand down, even briefly.

Smiling and laughter offer the body simple, physical signals that safety is present. In those moments, tension eases, breathing deepens and the nervous system is gently reminded that it can loosen its grip and return to balance.

These signals do not need to be dramatic or constant; even brief moments can shift the internal environment in meaningful ways.

Over time, those moments accumulate. A nervous system that regularly receives cues of ease becomes more flexible and resilient. Sleep begins to deepen, digestion settles, recovery improves and energy returns with greater consistency.

Regeneration unfolds through repeated signals that tell the body it is supported, connected and allowed to rest. Sometimes that signal is a shared joke, a spontaneous laugh or a smile that spreads without effort. These small expressions of lightness are not trivial; they are biological invitations for the body to repair, recalibrate and remember how to feel at ease again.

Regeneration in practice

Imagine you twist your ankle stepping off a kerb. In a nervous system stuck in a defensive state, stress chemistry stays high for much longer than the injury requires. The inflammatory response becomes amplified, the tissues stay irritated for longer and the brain interprets signals from the area as higher priority, which means you feel more discomfort than the injury actually warrants.

In a nervous system that resets more easily, the shift into repair mode happens far sooner. Inflammation rises and falls on schedule, the repair chemistry activates on time, and the tissue begins recovering without delay.

Now scale that across every organ and system. A steady nervous system improves the timing and accuracy of every repair process, which is why it sits at the heart of regeneration.

Trauma's Footprint - The Long-Term Cost

Unresolved trauma isn't "just in your head". It's a full-body experience that rewires how you operate, even when you think you've "moved on".

- **Structural:** Chronic stress reshapes key brain areas: the hippocampus (memory and learning) can shrink, the amygdala (fear centre) can become overactive, and the prefrontal cortex (logic, planning, impulse control) can lose efficiency. This creates a brain primed for hyper-vigilance and reactive decision-making rather than calm problem-solving.
- **Hormonal:** The stress hormones cortisol and adrenaline, meant for short bursts of survival, stay elevated. That constant chemical drip weakens muscles, disrupts sleep and throws metabolism off track, making fat easier to gain and harder to lose.
- **Immune:** The immune system shifts into a low-grade inflammatory state, like an engine running too hot. This increases the risk of autoimmune issues, allergies and even certain cancers.

- **Somatic:** Trauma doesn't just live in thoughts; it anchors itself in the body. Tight shoulders, clenched jaws, shallow breathing and gut discomfort become the "new normal". Over time, these patterns limit oxygenation, reduce mobility and disrupt digestion and nutrient absorption.

Left unchecked for years, these changes speed up biological ageing, raise cardiovascular risk and suppress the body's regenerative systems, including tissue repair, hormone balance and even the health of your microbiome.

The good news is that neuroplasticity, targeted movement, breathwork and recalibrating the autonomic nervous system can reverse much of this. You can't erase the past, but you can stop it dictating your future health.

The Regeneration Link

The nervous system is plastic. That means it can adapt, rewire and recover, even after years of being stuck in survival mode. The goal isn't to live in permanent calm but to restore flexibility, the ability to move between sympathetic and parasympathetic states as needed.

Practical regeneration starts with noticing your default state. Are you living mostly in fight, flight, freeze or fawn? Once you know that, you can start using targeted tools: breathwork, movement, sensory engagement or social support, to expand your range and recover your balance.

Regeneration Now - What Science (and Vanity) Already Offers

Regeneration once sounded like science fiction. Now it's in hospitals, wellness clinics, spas and the vitamin aisle of your local supermarket. Some of it is grounded in serious science, some of it is marketing dressed in a lab coat and some sits in the messy middle: promising but not yet fully proven. Still, all of it points to one truth: your body is not static, it can be coaxed, nudged and in some cases tricked into repair.

Stem Cells - The Master Builders

Stem cells are the body's master builders, capable of becoming the tissue that needs repair, whether that is bone, cartilage, nerve or muscle. In childhood these cells are abundant and responsive, which is why injuries heal quickly. By midlife the pool is smaller and slower to wake, and that is one of the reasons recovery feels sluggish and niggles linger longer than they used to.

Alongside your natural stem cells sit mesenchymal stem cells / Medicinal Signalling Cells (MSC), a group involved in structural repair, immune modulation and inflammation control. Their behaviour changes with age as well, and the signals that guide them become quieter unless the surrounding environment supports their activity.

- **Orthopaedic clinics** are already trialling MSC cell injections for arthritis and joint degeneration. In some cases, patients have avoided or postponed knee replacements for years.
- **Sports medicine** uses platelet-rich plasma (PRP), not pure stem cells but a cousin therapy that concentrates your own repair factors to accelerate healing in tendons and ligaments.
- **Longevity research** is exploring ways to "wake up" dormant stem cells. Fasting, high-intensity exercise, cold immersion and heat therapy have all been shown to trigger new stem cell activity. You don't need to fly to a Swiss clinic to switch them on, though people will happily charge you as if you do.

The limits: Stem cell therapies remain expensive, experimental and unevenly regulated. Results vary widely, which is why responsible clinicians treat them as promising but not guaranteed.

Even without injections, lifestyle practices that nudge the system through controlled stress and recovery still activate many of the same pathways.

The point is not to chase a single therapy but to create an internal environment where these master builders can work with more precision.

Collagen - The Scaffolding

If stem cells are the builders, collagen is the scaffolding. It's the protein mesh that keeps skin elastic, joints smooth, bones resilient and tendons strong. By your late 20s, collagen production starts to decline. By midlife, you feel it: wrinkles, stiffness, brittle nails and aching joints.

- **Collagen supplements** (powders, peptides, gummies, drinks) are booming. Hydrolysed collagen peptides are small enough to be absorbed, and studies suggest benefits for skin elasticity, joint pain and bone health.
- **Vitamin C** is the unsung partner. Collagen synthesis literally cannot happen without it. Forgetting vitamin C while taking collagen powder is like hiring builders but never giving them nails.
- **Lifestyle factors** matter. UV exposure, smoking, high sugar intake and chronic stress all accelerate collagen breakdown. You can't out-supplement self-sabotage.

The limits: Not all collagen is created equal. Some powders are bulked out, underdosed, or poorly absorbed and no matter the marketing, it's not a miracle in a scoop. Collagen works best as part of a broader repair protocol.

Botox and Fillers - Quick Cosmetic Fixes

Botox is the opposite of regeneration. It works by paralysing muscles, so skin appears smoother. Fillers puff out wrinkles or lost volume by injecting gel-like substances under the skin. Both can make the surface look "refreshed", but underneath, nothing has been rebuilt.

To put it bluntly, Botox is like decorating over damp.

That doesn't make these fixes useless; confidence matters and for some people, these treatments deliver exactly what they want, but they are surface-level solutions. They don't improve collagen, stem cells, or nervous system repair. If anything, over-reliance can distract from addressing the deeper biology that actually governs ageing.

Pulling It Together

Regeneration is already here but it's fragmented. You can inject stem cells, scoop collagen, swallow amino acids, paralyse wrinkles or sit in a cryotherapy chamber. The question isn't whether it works, as much of it does, but how deep it goes. Do you want the surface painted, or the foundations rebuilt?

That choice is the difference between cosmetic intervention and true regeneration.

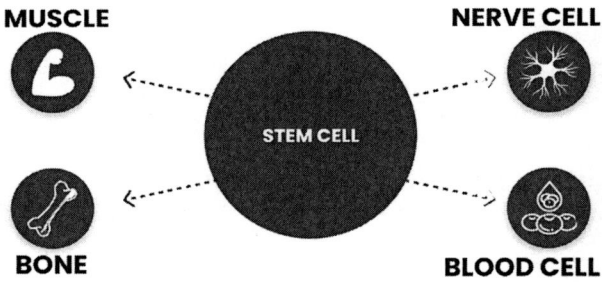

The Next Phase of Biological Regeneration

Here is what I see when I look across the field right now. On one end you have serious labs pushing stem cells, gene switches and tissue engineering. On the other you have cosmetic quick fixes that smooth the surface while the structure underneath stays the same. In the middle sits a maze of supplements, wearables and wellness rituals that often work but rarely talk to each other. The biology is not the problem, the lack of integration is.

That is why I decided to engineer a system rather than add another pill, cream or class. The body runs on signals, and if we can coordinate the right signals at the right time, the system regenerates. Simple idea, hard engineering.

Regeneration Next - Where It's Heading

Right now, regeneration is a patchwork quilt. A bit of stem cell here, a collagen scoop there, a handful of supplements and maybe a Botox top-up if you fancy wallpapering the cracks. But the future is not more patches, it's a combination of getting

Pillar 3 - Biology: You Are Not a Machine

the timing, the signals and the delivery right so the body does the heavy lifting itself.

Stem cells and reprogramming
Stem cell banking will become the ultimate rainy-day fund. Instead of saving cash for your kids to blow on a gap year, you'll be saving your own cells so your knees can still handle a flight of stairs at 70. Beyond that, labs are already trialling "partial reprogramming", teaching your older cells to behave younger without sending them rogue. It sounds like science fiction but then again, so did keyhole surgery once.

Beyond capsules
The supplement aisle is currently expensive urine insurance: you swallow, you hope, but most of it ends up down the toilet. The future is smarter delivery: patches that drip-feed nutrients through your skin, nasal sprays and inhaled mists that hit your bloodstream in seconds, and microneedle films that bypass digestion altogether. It's not what you take, it's how and when your biology receives it.

Environments For Success – Regen by Design
Ancient healers used heat, cold, scent, rhythm, darkness and pressure to shift state. Modern clinics use red and near infrared light for mitochondria, far infrared heat for relaxation and blood flow, magnetic fields to nudge cellular charge and sound to slow the brain out of threat mode. None of this replaces foundations, it turns good foundations into faster outcomes.

The next phase is closed loop. Sensors read your state in real time: light and heat and sound adjust automatically, and supplementation is delivered through skin or breath at the exact moment your biology is most ready to use it. This is engineering working with you.

AI and timing

Wearables today give you bedtime guilt ("you only had 5 hours 42 minutes, do better!"). Tomorrow's systems will actually tell you when to move, eat, or sleep for maximum repair. AI doesn't care about averages; it cares about your biology in real time: *protein now, stretch later, lights out at 10.07*. It sounds bossy but so does your satnav and we all still use it. Tools like MAI-Motion exist for exactly this reason. Motion is data. Data becomes feedback. Feedback becomes control.

Whole-body transformation

This is the horizon; not fixing one broken part but preventing them all from breaking. Imagine full-body programmes combining stem cells, targeted light and heat, nutrition through patches and sprays and data-driven timing. It's not about turning you into Wolverine, it's about recalibrating the system so joints, skin, brain and immunity all stay younger for longer.

The Regen PhD Pod and Biology

When creating the Pod I was aware that your body already has the systems for repair: stem cells that rebuild, hormones that signal, immune cells that clean up and tissues that lay down fresh collagen. The problem is they are easily disrupted by stress, poor timing and background noise.

Whilst the Pod does not replace those systems, it creates the conditions for them to work the way they should. Heat, light, vibration and calm signals lower interference so biology can switch back into repair mode. In practice that means cells release more energy, hormones follow their natural rhythm, the immune system clears damage more effectively and tissues have the environment they need to rebuild.

The beauty is that I did not reinvent the wheel, I just combined the good stuff out there and made it easy and deliverable or accessible. This is not new science; it is practical science.

In biology, the right signal at the right time makes the difference between decline and repair. The Pod is built to provide those signals in a coordinated way, so regeneration becomes predictable instead of left to chance.

The horizon

Stem cell banking will move from specialist to standard. Partial cellular reprogramming will shift from papers to protocols with strict safeguards. Absorption based supplementation will beat capsules. AI will run the timing, but the rules will stay human. Eat real food. Sleep in darkness. Keep regular hours. Move with load and rhythm. Protect the nervous system from living on a hair trigger. Measure what matters. Change one variable at a time. Keep what works.

The forest you carry inside you does not need a miracle, it needs conditions. The industry is finally learning to provide them and that is the future. Not a new you invented by a lab, but your system rebuilt by signals it has trusted for thousands of years, delivered with the precision we can now build.

Chapter Summary

This chapter explored how regeneration is sustained over time, not through isolated fixes but through living systems that communicate, adapt and respond continuously. Biology is the layer that keeps everything working together: digestion, hormones, rhythms, sleep and the nervous system, all trading signals moment by moment.

You learned why the body behaves less like a machine and more like an ecosystem. Changes in one area ripple across the whole system. Stress alters digestion. Sleep timing reshapes hormone release. Gut microbes influence immunity, mood and recovery.

The body can compensate for imbalance for a while, but when signals stay noisy or mistimed, strain appears as fatigue, pain, weight change, disrupted sleep or emotional instability.

This chapter showed how to work with biology rather than override it. Instead of chasing symptoms, the focus is on recognising patterns, reducing background noise and using simple, repeatable inputs to restore coordination. Early signs such as energy on waking, digestion, body temperature, mood stability and recovery speed matter long before pathology appears on a scan.

Biology also framed why trauma and midlife shifts change the rules. A nervous system shaped by prolonged stress adapts for protection, not repair. Hormonal transitions alter sleep, joint comfort, tissue recovery and energy regulation. In both cases, regeneration depends on creating conditions the body recognises as safe, predictable and supportive, rather than forcing performance.

Across digestion, hormones, rhythm, sleep and nervous system function, the same principle repeated: timing matters. When signals arrive at the right moment, repair becomes efficient. When timing drifts, systems work harder for less return.

The outcome of well-regulated biology is not dramatic. It is reliable. Energy steadies. Sleep deepens. Digestion becomes unremarkable. Training supports recovery rather than depleting it. Pain resolves faster and emotional resilience becomes the default.

This is regeneration that holds, because the system underneath is working.

Practical Tools

You can't optimise what you don't measure. Sleep feels subjective but data can reveal patterns.

What to Track:
- **Duration:** How many hours do you sleep?
- **Efficiency:** Time asleep vs. time in bed.
- **Deep sleep/REM split:** More deep sleep = better repair, more REM = better memory / emotional balance.
- **Resting heart rate and HRV:** Lower resting heart rate and higher HRV = better recovery.

Tools:
- Oura Ring, Whoop, Apple Watch, or other wearables.
- Sleep diaries if you prefer low-tech: track bedtime, wake time, energy on waking and mood.

The Key: Don't obsess. Data is a compass, not a prison. Use it to spot patterns, e.g. *"I sleep deeper when I cut caffeine earlier"* or *"Alcohol always wrecks REM"*. Then act.

Pillar 3 - Biology: You Are Not a Machine

Here are some simple tables you can use to monitor your progress:

Date	Bedtime	Wake Time	Hours Slept	Energy (1-10)	Notes

Week	Avg. Hours	Best Night	Worst Night	Energy Trend	Notes

Nightly Wind-Down Checklist
- ☐ Lights dimmed, screens off (or blue light filter on)
- ☐ Breathing/stretching done (5–10 minutes)
- ☐ Notes/journal written, brain unloaded
- ☐ Warm drink/tea (chamomile, passionflower, or similar)
- ☐ Bedroom set: cool temperature, blackout curtains, calming scent
- ☐ Phone on silent/away from bed

Sleep Optimisation Checklist
- ☐ Bedroom is dark, cool and quiet (scents/sounds supportive)
- ☐ Wake time is consistent every day (even weekends)
- ☐ Pre-sleep ritual in place: lights dimmed, breathing/stretching, thoughts unloaded
- ☐ No caffeine after 2pm
- ☐ No heavy meals late at night
- ☐ Diet supports sleep (magnesium and tryptophan-rich foods)
- ☐ Sleep tracked (duration, quality, deep/REM balance, HRV if possible)
- ☐ Backup strategies planned: naps, yoga nidra, mindset reset

Backup Strategies - When Sleep Won't Come

Even with rituals and environments dialled in, life interferes. Here's how to recover when insomnia threatens.

1. **Naps**
   - 20 minutes = alertness boost.
   - 90 minutes = full cycle, deeper recovery.
   - Avoid late-afternoon naps if they delay night sleep.

2. **Yoga Nidra / NSDR (Non-Sleep Deep Rest)**
   - Guided meditations that mimic some of the brain and body benefits of sleep.
   - Reduces stress, restores focus and lowers cortisol.

3. **Mindset Shift**
   - Don't catastrophise a bad night. One poor night isn't the end.
   - Regeneration is cumulative. Stressing makes it worse.

Nervous System Reset Worksheet

We all move through fight, flight, freeze and fawn at different times. The question is: *Which one does your nervous system default to when under pressure?*

Your "default" is usually:
- The state you spend the most time in when stressed.
- The one you return to automatically, even without an obvious trigger.
- The pattern friends or family might notice before you do (you're always on edge / you always avoid things / you just shut down).

Below are common signs of each. Over the last month, tick the ones you've experienced most often, not just in big crises but in everyday life. Then see which column has the most ticks. That's probably your dominant mode.

Pillar 3 - Biology: You Are Not a Machine

Step 1 - Identify Your Default Mode

Tick any that apply over the last month:
Fight (confront & control)
- ☐ Frequent irritability or quick temper
- ☐ Jaw clenching or teeth grinding
- ☐ Feeling "wired" even when tired
- ☐ Digestive slowdown or reflux during stress

Flight (escape & avoid)
- ☐ Racing thoughts or inability to relax
- ☐ Avoiding calls, emails, or social contact
- ☐ Resting heart rate consistently over 85
- ☐ Digestive upset before events or deadlines

Freeze (immobilise)
- ☐ Procrastination despite wanting to act
- ☐ Numbness, zoning out, or mental fog
- ☐ Feeling heavy or stuck in one position
- ☐ Sleep doesn't restore energy

Fawn (appease & please)
- ☐ Automatically saying "yes" to requests
- ☐ Feeling unsafe when setting boundaries
- ☐ Mood depends heavily on others' approval
- ☐ Anxiety before potentially disappointing someone

Your main default mode(s): _____

Step 2 - Daily Reset Drill

If in Fight mode:
- 2 minutes of extended exhales (inhale for 4, exhale for 8)
- Drop shoulders, unclench jaw, massage temples

If in Flight mode:
- Brisk 5–10-minute walk
- Focus eyes on the horizon (shifts brain out of tunnel vision)

If in Freeze mode:
- Wiggle toes, tap fingers, slowly stretch arms
- Say out loud what you can see, hear and feel (sensory re-entry)

If in Fawn mode:
- Pause before saying "yes", tell the person you'll confirm later
- 3 slow breaths before responding in conversation

Step 3 – Three Minute Nervous System Check-In (Daily)

How to Check Your Resting Heart Rate
1. **Sit or lie down quietly** for at least 5 minutes.
2. **Find your pulse**, easiest is either:
   - **Wrist:** Place two fingers (not your thumb) on the inside of your opposite wrist, just below the base of your thumb.
   - **Neck:** Place two fingers gently on the side of your neck, just under your jawline.

3. **Count the beats for 30 seconds**, then multiply by 2. That's your beats per minute (BPM).
4. **Do it at the same time each day**, ideally first thing in the morning before you've had caffeine or done any activity.
5. **Typical ranges:**
    - 60–80 BPM = average adult range
    - Athletes or those with high fitness can be in the 40–60 range
    - Consistently above 85 BPM at rest may indicate that your nervous system is staying in a heightened activation state.

Once a day, note:
- **Heart rate:** _____ bpm
- **Breathing:** Shallow / Normal / Deep
- **Muscle tension:** High / Medium / Low
- **Mood:** Calm / Alert / Anxious / Low
- **Dominant mode right now:** Fight / Flight / Freeze / Fawn

Step 4 - Vagus Nerve Conditioning (Pick 1–2 daily)
- Humming for 2–3 minutes
- Gargling for 30 seconds
- Splashing cold water on the face or cold shower
- Singing loudly to a song you enjoy
- Laughter (real or even "fake it until it becomes real")

Step 5 - Weekly Review

Which mode showed up most? _____

Did recovery feel faster compared to last week? Yes / No

Which habit felt easiest to stick with? _____

Next week's focus: _____

Summary: Your nervous system learns through repetition, this worksheet isn't about "fixing" yourself overnight; it's about creating a safe, consistent environment where your body relearns how to move between states.
That's regeneration in real time.

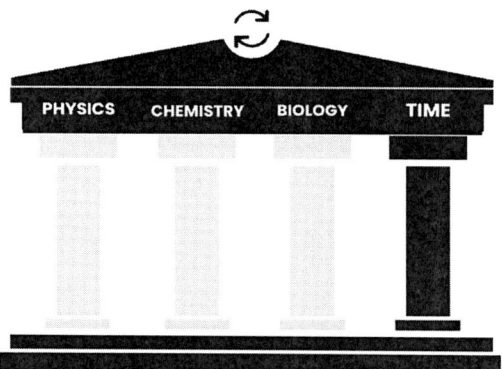

Pillar 4 - Time: The Missing Variable

"You can't force biology to hurry – but you can stop wasting time on the wrong things."

"A man who dares to waste one hour of time has not discovered the value of life."

Charles Darwin.

Time - The Hidden Force

We spend our lives obsessing over inputs. Counting calories, tracking steps, buying supplements we can't even pronounce. Downloading sleep apps to tell us what we already know – we're tired. We cram more into our diaries and then complain there aren't enough hours in the day.

Yet here's the question almost nobody asks: *what's time itself doing to your body?*

That's the bit we miss.

Physics gave us the frame. Chemistry gave us the ingredients. Biology gave us the living machine. But none of those pillars mean a thing without the one element nobody escapes: time.

Ignore time and you don't just miss progress, you lose it. Miss a healing window and it's gone. Not delayed or paused, it's gone. Delay a decision and you're not standing still; you're rolling backwards while pretending you're "waiting it out".

People act like time is neutral, but it isn't. Waiting is expensive as it compounds everything, it takes little cracks and turns them into structural failure. Time is the invisible hand pushing biology forwards or dragging it down.

Unlike money, you can't earn it back; there's no refund, no credit line. Once it's spent, it's irreplaceable.

Healing Clocks You Can't Cheat

Every biological process runs on timing. That's not philosophy but hardwired physiology.

Break a bone and there's a script your body follows: inflammation, soft callus, hard callus, remodelling. Each stage depends on the last. Miss the stability window in those first few weeks and the fracture doesn't knit straight. You live with that forever, or you go back in for the fun of having it re-broken and re-set, which is no fun for anyone.

Tear a ligament and collagen fibres rush in to knit the gap. Do the right things then and they line up like soldiers: strong, elastic, ready for action. Push too early or wait too long and those fibres tangle into scar tissue. Scar tissue doesn't stretch; it frays. You don't get the neat elastic band back; you get a rope with knots in it.

Even at the micro level, the body runs on clocks. Train hard and your muscle fibres open a door for repair but only for a set window. Protein synthesis peaks for hours and growth hormone pulses at night. Miss those signals and you're not just wasting effort; you're training for nothing. You sweated for it, but the repair crew was off shift. No cells, no gain.

That's the truth people don't like – healing isn't infinite, it's opportunity-based. Windows open, windows close and they don't hang around for for you to be ready.

The Illusion of Neutral Waiting

People think waiting is harmless. They see a delay as "just time" but in biology, waiting is never neutral. A six-month delay isn't just six months of pain, it's six months of altered movement, of compensation patterns building, of inflammation embedding into tissues, and of pain pathways wiring deeper into the nervous system.

Think of your body like a dashboard full of warning lights. Pain is the red flash telling you something's wrong. Ignore it and the problem doesn't pause politely it compounds.

- A limp you "put up with" throws your hip and spine out of alignment.
- A stiff shoulder you ignore begins to freeze surrounding joints.
- A digestive issue you brush aside sends immune signals that ripple through your whole system.

Waiting is active damage

Warning Lights and Compounding Damage

Here's how it really works. Your body gives you early signals: a flicker of knee pain on the stairs, a shoulder that clicks when you reach overhead or fatigue that comes earlier than it used to.

Ignore those warnings and you're not "saving time". You're compounding the problem. That ache becomes altered movement. That altered movement stresses another joint. That stress creates inflammation. Eventually you're not dealing with one problem, you're dealing with five.

Think of it like driving on a spare tyre. For the first few days it seems fine, but a week later the car feels slightly off, a month later the suspension's wearing unevenly, and six months down the line you're looking at alignment issues, tired shocks and extra strain on the bearings. That's not one problem anymore, all because you didn't replace the wheel immediately.

Biology works the same way. Ignore the problem and you're not staying where you, you're quietly stacking up interest on the damage, and it always comes due.

Time as a Currency

We're conditioned to think of money as the ultimate currency, but money can be earned back, every day you spend in pain that could have been resolved is time permanently withdrawn from your life and once it's gone, it doesn't refill.

That's why the question isn't "can I afford to act now?" The real question is: "how much time am I willing to throw away?"

Why This Pillar Exists

Physics taught you that structure matters, Chemistry showed you inputs and Biology explained the living network. Time is the frame that makes them all work or fail.

This section will demonstrate that regeneration isn't just about what you do. It's about *when you do it*.

Why Healing Has Non-Negotiable Windows

People love to think of the body as forgiving. Twist something, strain something, push through and eventually it'll sort itself out, or so the story goes. But your body isn't forgiving. It runs to a schedule older than civilisation, written into the chemistry of every cell. Healing phases open, they do their work and then they shut.

That's why we need to stop pretending we can bargain with the body's clock. You can haggle with a builder to shift a deadline. You can reschedule a meeting, move a flight or delay an exam but your body can't be negotiated with. When the repair cycle has passed, no amount of willpower, supplements or clever hacks can re-open it.

These biological deadlines run through every layer of us: muscles, nerves, organs, even the way we age.

Micro-Timelines Inside the Body

The moment tissue is injured a whole emergency crew rushes to the scene. We see inflammation as a negative thing but in reality it's search and rescue. Within minutes, white blood cells swarm in, clearing debris, killing bacteria and releasing cytokines that call for backup. Platelets clot, forming a temporary barrier. Fibroblasts arrive, laying down scaffolding for new tissue.

Pillar 4 - Time: The Missing Variable

That early inflammatory surge is essential. Shut it down too aggressively, say, by drowning yourself in anti-inflammatories and you fire the clean-up crew before the job is done. What's left is half-cleared tissue, sluggish healing and a mess the body has to patch over with scar tissue. That's why some people "never feel quite right" after what should have been a minor injury. They interfered with the first critical phase of repair.

Inflammation isn't the bad guy, (out-of-control, chronic inflammation is) but those early hours and days are the biological equivalent of emergency services arriving at a crash site. You wouldn't send them away while the car was still burning, but by swallowing ibuprofen and carrying on, you're doing just that.

Muscles and the Myth of "Catching Up Later"

The same principle applies to muscles. After you train, muscle fibres are primed for repair. Protein synthesis surges for hours, growth hormone pulses at night, not whenever you happen to collapse into bed.

Athletes know this because they're coached effectively and taught what their body needs. That's why they obsess over meal timing, post-training recovery shakes and sleep hygiene. They're not fussy; they're exploiting biology's repair cycles while the system is listening.

Contrast that with the average person who shrugs and says, "I'll catch up later". There is no "later". If you miss the surge, you miss the adaptation. The training session becomes punishment instead of progress. A few beers with friends after your workout has a negative effect; you're left sore but no stronger.

Your body doesn't give you rollover minutes like a phone contract.

Ligaments and the Scar Tissue Trap

Ligaments are even more unforgiving. Tear one and collagen fibres rush in to knit the structure. In the first few weeks, those fibres are like fresh dough: pliable and responsive. With the right load at the right time, they align neatly, forming strong elastic bands.

Leave it too long or stress it too soon and the fibres tangle into scar tissue. Scar tissue is like Velcro: stiff, messy, and always catching where it shouldn't. Once it sets, you can't knead it back into rope. That opportunity for clean repair is gone.

Patients often ask, "Can you loosen this scar up?" The honest answer is no. You missed the chance when the fibres were still arranging themselves. That's not me or your consultant being cruel, that's biology's version of "deadline passed".

Nerves: Use It or Lose It

Nerve healing is slower still: a millimetre a day. That's about as fast as your fingernails grow. Worse, nerves have a strict use-it-or-lose-it rule. Fail to stimulate them in time and the pathways fade, muscles waiting for signals atrophy and sensation doesn't return.

This is why the first few weeks after a stroke are so critical. The nervous system is in a rare state of plasticity, desperate to rewire, miss that period and the reorganisation sets in. You can still make gains later, but you'll never have the same chance to reclaim lost function.

The same goes for chronic pain. Let acute pain run for too long and the brain learns it. Neurons fire more easily, pain signals amplify and what began as a sprain becomes a permanent part of your nervous system. You didn't just miss a window; you taught your brain to keep the pain switched on.

Pain is like an alarm, but alarms are supposed to turn off once you act. Leave them blaring and eventually your nervous system rewires itself to the sound.

The brain learns to recognise threat. If a movement, place or time of day was paired with pain, your amygdala remembers and prepares you to guard. Sometimes it produces the sensation by itself. This is often the case where trauma is involved. None of this means pain is "in your head", it means the system designed to protect you adapts and sometimes it over-protects. The fix is not just pills; it's graded exposure, sleep, stress control, nutrition and well-timed rehab that rewrites those circuits. None of these may be needed if the original problem is dealt with in the correct way.

Ageing: The Longest Clock of All

Then there's ageing, the ultimate, universal timetable. Every year, telomeres shorten, stem cells thin out, repair systems grow less efficient. That doesn't mean decline happens at the same pace for everyone however, it does mean you can't leave it until "later".

The choices you make in your thirties and forties – sleep, exercise, diet, stress – decide what kind of fifties, sixties and seventies you'll have. Think of it like compound interest. Start early and the benefits snowball, start late and you're running uphill with a shrinking repair budget.

Ageing is delayed healing in slow motion. The repair cycles get narrower, the thresholds lower, the stakes higher. Respect time early and you change what ageing feels like, ignore it and you're forced to live with biology's late-payment fees.

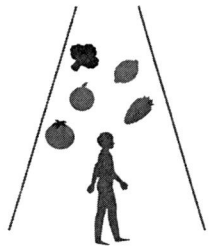

Regeneration

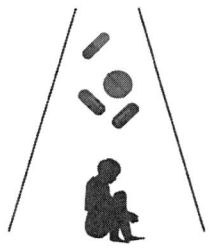

Deregeneration

The Orchestra in Your Cells

Here's the part where I get excited, because the precision of it is extraordinary. Every cell in your body is running on molecular clocks. Genes switch on and off in 24-hour rhythms. Hormones surge and dip with the light. Immune cells patrol more aggressively at night.

It's like a global orchestra playing a score millions of years old. Bones, muscles, nerves, organs – every section has its cue. Get it right and the music is seamless; miss it and you can't just ask the orchestra to start again, the moment has passed.

People often say to me, "But surely I can make up for lost time?" That's not how orchestras work. You don't clap your hands and tell the violins to replay their entrance because you were late. Biology moves forwards whether you're ready or not.

Culture: Soldiering On and Waiting It Out

It seems that, especially in Britain, we love the myth of "soldiering on". We limp through work, shrug off back pain, ignore lumps and pat ourselves on the back for not making a fuss. Biology isn't impressed, it doesn't hand out medals for endurance.

Contrast that with elite athletes: they stop, they scan, they treat, because they know what delay costs. Their careers depend on respecting timing. Meanwhile, the rest of us often treat our only body with less urgency than they treat a hamstring.

This is a cultural problem. We are conditioned to the busyness of life – many of us have become workaholics either through passion for what we do, or necessity to cover the cost of living. The thought of stopping is terrifying: *"How do I pay my bills, what if I get fired, what if I don't get that promotion…?"* What if you don't stop? The body has a way of forcing you and usually by that point it's far worse and takes far longer to come back.

The Practical Lesson

So, here's the blunt truth:
- Every tissue, every system, has critical periods where repair is possible.
- Miss them and the chance doesn't come round again.
- Waiting isn't neutral. It's active damage, compounding while you tell yourself you're "being sensible".
- You are expendable and life will go on if you take time to heal.

You don't need to obsess over every molecule in your body, but you do need to respect the clocks.

Practical Toolkit: REPAIR

R - Respect the alarm
- Pain, swelling, or sudden weakness are not "niggles", they're your red warnings.
- Don't mute them with painkillers and pride. Note *when it started, what triggered it and whether it's getting worse.*

E - Early action
- The first 2–6 weeks are decisive. Small injuries can either heal clean or become lifelong problems in this phase.
- Seek assessment sooner rather than later. Even a basic plan (rest, ice/heat, movement guidance) keeps you aligned with biology's repair cycle.

P - Protective movement
- Total rest stiffens and weakens; over movement tears fibres apart. The sweet spot is *guided, progressive movement.*
- If you're not sure, stay on the side of controlled mobility, gentle stretching, basic load and short walks.

A - Adequate fuel
- Protein within hours of stress, anti-inflammatory foods (not pills), hydration and micronutrients all feed the repair machinery.
- Sleep is non-negotiable. Growth hormone surges at night; miss it and you blunt healing.

I - Intervene before chronicity
- If pain persists beyond normal healing time (6–12 weeks), don't "wait it out". That's when the nervous system starts to learn pain.
- Intervention might mean physiotherapy, graded activity, stress reduction or pain re-education.

R - Remember ageing
- The older you are, the less flexible the timelines. Collagen stiffens, stem cells slow and recovery phases shrink.
- That doesn't mean giving up; it means acting faster. What you delay at 30 costs you months; what you delay at 60 can cost you years.

 One-line mantra: *If you respect the REPAIR cycle, your body regenerates.*

How Delay Compounds into Damage

We like to believe waiting is safe. Waiting feels polite, reasonable, even cautious.

"If I don't poke it, maybe it won't get worse."

Here's the truth: in biology, delay isn't a pause button, it's like petrol on the fire.

What makes this worse is that everyone already knows this. Nobody ignores the oil light on their car for a year or watches a crack zig-zag down the wall of their house and thinks they will leave it for a few months. Yet when it's about their own body, sometimes people act as if time is infinite and biology will wait politely.

It won't.

The Compound-Interest Problem

Biology works a bit like finance. Time isn't passive; it compounds problems.

Ignore back pain for a fortnight and your muscles tighten to protect you. Leave it for a year and your hips, knees and posture have all reorganised to accommodate the pain. The back isn't the only problem anymore; your whole framework is off.

Delay treating a knee injury and you don't just damage the cartilage further; you overload the opposite knee. Before you know it, both sides hurt and you've doubled the problem.

Put off surgery long enough and scar tissue weaves in, making the eventual procedure longer, riskier and less effective.

It's never just the original problem, time adds interest.

Harsh Truth

People tell me: *"Oh, I didn't want to bother anyone. I thought it might get better."*

I want to say: *like anything else that goes wrong, it won't always get better on its own if you just hope that it will.*

Real-Life Example

Margaret was 68 when she came to me, though her walk made her look closer to 85. Her right hip was so stiff she had to swing her whole body around to move the leg forwards. Getting onto the consultation couch took three attempts, each one punctuated with a wince and an apology, as though the pain was somehow her fault.

The story was depressingly familiar. Five years earlier she'd felt "a bit of stiffness in the mornings". Nothing major, she told herself. It eased once she got moving, so she carried on. A year later she was limping on supermarket runs but she put it down to "just ageing". By the third year, she was in enough pain to see her GP, who put her on a waiting list. She sighed, shrugged and decided to wait it out.

Here's the problem with waiting lists: time doesn't stand still while you're on them. Margaret's cartilage wore thinner, her bone hardened and deformed under pressure and her muscles tightened into protective knots. Her spine twisted subtly to take the load, then her knees and ankles started to ache. By the time she was called in for surgery, the joint hadn't just deteriorated, it had collapsed.

In Margaret's case though, delay had another sting. She was post-menopause. The drop in oestrogen that comes with menopause isn't just about hot flushes, it accelerates bone thinning and joint degeneration. What might have been a slow decline in her fifties became a rapid landslide in her sixties. Every year of delay carried more weight than the year before.

So, by 68 she wasn't just dealing with a bad hip. She was dealing with compounded age-related muscle loss, stiffer collagen, reduced healing capacity and the hormonal legacy of menopause. Biology had stacked the deck against her and time had been the dealer.

Operating on a hip that far gone is a different beast. Instead of a neat replacement, we faced distorted anatomy, scar tissue and a recovery measured not in months but in years. The surgery took longer, the risks were higher and the outcome was permanently limited. Margaret could walk again, yes, but she would never get back the ease of movement she might have had if we'd caught it five years earlier.

When I asked why she'd waited, she looked embarrassed. "I thought it would get better, and I didn't want to make a fuss." That phrase, *didn't want to make a fuss*, could be carved onto the gravestone of half the preventable disability in this country.

Here's the real point: if Margaret had acted sooner, we could have replaced the joint before collapse. Her gait would have been preserved, her spine spared and her independence protected. Instead, delay compounded into damage. She didn't just lose cartilage; she lost years of quality life, and the compounding effect of age and menopause meant those years were the very years she needed most.

The cruel irony? Margaret was super-efficient and made sure she checked the batteries in her smoke alarm, paid her bills on time and had her car booked in for annual services. However, with her hip screaming every step, she thought silence and stoicism were the answer.

Inside the Body: Where Delay Becomes Damage

We've talked about hips, backs and joints: the things people notice when they creak. But the most dangerous clocks are the ones you can't hear. Almost every system in your body has its own countdown and most of them don't send polite reminders. By the time symptoms shout, the damage is already baked in.

Heart & Blood Vessels: Seconds Matter

In a **stroke**, 1.9 million neurons die every minute without blood flow. "Time is brain cells" isn't a slogan, it's genuine fact. Delayed treatment means entire abilities vanish: speech, movement and memory.

In a **heart attack**, cardiologists say "time is muscle". Once heart muscle dies, it's replaced by scar tissue which doesn't beat. Every delay turns a reversible blockage into permanent heart failure.

Liver: The Unknown Collapse

The liver is a master of endurance. It can lose 70% of its function before you notice a thing. People with early fatty liver disease feel "fine". That's the trap. Delay turns fat into inflammation, inflammation into fibrosis and fibrosis into cirrhosis. By then the organ's architecture is collapsing in on itself.

Act early with better diet, alcohol reduction and weight management can reverse it. If you wait too long your only options may be transplant lists and lifelong complications.

Kidneys: Nothing Until They Crash

Kidneys compensate so well that they can lose most of their function before you feel anything is wrong. Blood tests can look normal, you can feel "just tired", but the damage continues in the background.

That is why kidney disease is so dangerous; the lack of symptoms hides the decline. If you carry risks such as diabetes or high blood pressure, or you are aged over sixty or on long term painkiller use, waiting for symptoms is not a safe strategy because the signals can arrive late. Regular blood and urine tests are essential, creating a pattern you monitor over time.

When kidneys fail, your choices narrow to dialysis or a transplant. Acting early keeps you in control.

Lungs: Breath on Borrowed Time

With Chronic Obstructive Pulmonary Disease (COPD), every cigarette is time ticking away. Damage stacks until one day you notice you're breathless on the stairs. By then, you've already lost lung capacity you're never getting back.

With pneumonia, wait too long for antibiotics or oxygen and the lungs stiffen with fibrosis. Survivors often live with permanent breathlessness because they thought they'd "ride it out". Breath is time. Lose one and you lose the other.

Pancreas & Diabetes: The Long Game

Type 2 diabetes it stalks you daily. People often delay the lifestyle tweaks, the meds and the check-ups. Every delay is another microvascular hit:
- Eyes → retinopathy, blindness.
- Kidneys → nephropathy, failure.
- Nerves → neuropathy, ulcers, amputations.

The cruel part is that early action can literally stop these from happening. Wait long enough and you swap "manageable condition" for "permanent complication".

Then there's acute pancreatitis. That's a horror film. Delay treatment and the pancreas starts digesting itself which should be grotesque enough on its own to move you to action.

Bones & Joints: The Compound Fracture of Time

Osteoporosis accelerates after menopause. The first 5–10 years are when bone density falls off a cliff. Delayed intervention, strength work, calcium or meds means fractures are inevitable. A hip fracture at 70 isn't just a broken bone; it's often the start of the end for independence.

Arthritis? Not just "wear and tear". A delay in offloading the stress or building strength and cartilage disappears faster. It's worth noting that cartilage doesn't grow back. By the time it's bone grinding on bone, the only solution left is replacement. This in itself is terribly hard if there is little muscle to work with as you get titanium on bone which can be just as painful.

Bones have deadlines. Ignore them and you don't just get aches, you get rods, plates, scars and a surgeon's signature on your skeleton.

Eyes: Vision on a Clock

Glaucoma progresses with no early warning. It damages the optic nerve fibre by fibre without pain or blur and many people only notice it once parts of their peripheral vision have already disappeared. Those losses are permanent because the damaged fibres do not regenerate. Early testing is the only way to catch it.

Macular degeneration works in a similar way. You may see clearly in the early stages, yet the underlying changes continue. Diet, targeted treatment and lifestyle support can slow the decline, but once central blind spots appear, they do not reverse.

The mistake many people make is relying on how their vision feels. Clear sight does not tell you what is happening to your retina or your optic nerve. Glasses correct blur, not disease. Proper eye examinations are the only way to detect these conditions before the damage becomes irreversible.

Whilst eye tests can be expensive, your sight is priceless.

Immune System & Cancer: Deadlines You Can't See

Cancer is one of the clearest examples of why time matters. The difference between catching it early and finding it late isn't a small detail, it can be life or death. Stage 1 bowel cancer, caught early, has around a 90% five-year survival rate. Stage 4, after it's spread, drops closer to 10%.

The tumour isn't waiting while you decide if you're "ready" to deal with it. Cells divide, relentlessly and by the time you're aware enough of your symptoms, the window for the best outcomes may already be behind you.

Sepsis is even more unforgiving. It doesn't run on months or years, it runs on hours. Every delay in antibiotics increases the chance of organ failure and death. What started as "a bit of a fever" can become a fight for life by the end of the day.

I'm not trying to scare anyone; I just want to be very clear on the importance of seeking help. With cancer and sepsis, delay doesn't just make recovery harder, sometimes it takes recovery off the table completely.

Age: The Universal Multiplier

Every clock ticks louder with age. The same six-month delay at 30 costs you discomfort, at 60, it costs independence, at 80, it can cost your life.

Yet, we shrug and mutter, *"It's probably nothing."* We wait. Waiting is the biggest accelerant of damage you'll ever meet.

Psychology of Delay

Why do some people do this? Mainly because delay feels safe, like you're "not making it worse". In reality, delay is a decision. Choosing not to act is still an action and in biology it's almost always the wrong one.

There's also fear. People avoid doctors because they don't want bad news but refusing to receive it doesn't change the facts. That's like leaving your credit card bill unopened because you don't want to see the numbers. The interest still runs and the debt still grows.

Clinical Stories

This isn't theory. I've seen it every week of my career.
- A shoulder niggle ignored for six months stiffened into a frozen joint. That pulled the neck out of alignment, which then dragged the spine into the problem. One small delay created three new issues.
- A runner who "pushed through" shin pain ended up with a stress fracture. The compensation wrecked her gait so badly her hips and back joined the party.

- A patient who delayed a knee replacement "just a bit longer". By the time we operated, the joint had collapsed, the bone was warped and the outcome was permanently limited.

Every single case could have been simpler, shorter and less damaging if treated on time. Delay accelerates damage, always.

Irreversible Time

Here's something interesting. In physics, time can be reversible and equations run both ways. You can rewind the tape, reverse the reaction, rerun the maths backwards and it still works. In biology? Forget it, biology is one-way traffic

That's why waiting is so dangerous. Some people act as if their body is in storage, "I'll deal with this later, it'll still be fresh". No. Delay is like leaving milk past its use-by date: it doesn't just sit there waiting for you to be ready; it curdles and once it's sour, no amount of wishful thinking makes it drinkable again.

Younger Patients: The Hidden Delay

It's tempting to think that undervaluing health is something that happens in later life, when bodies creak, joints grind and people resign themselves to the phrase "it's just age". In my clinic though, some of the most worrying delays aren't from patients in their seventies or eighties. They're from people in their thirties and forties, sometimes even younger.

Why? They believe they're too young for anything serious.

This mindset is one of the most dangerous traps I see. A pulled hamstring at 35, a nagging shoulder after a gym session, a stiff hip after a football match: all of these get dismissed. Patients tell themselves they'll "walk it off", that it's "normal", or that their body will "sort itself out". Painkillers go in, a bit of stretching gets done and life carries on. Outwardly, nothing has changed. Inwardly, biology is already moving in the wrong direction.

The Illusion of Youth

Younger patients often believe they have time on their side. They expect their bodies to bounce back because that's what they did at 20. They mistake resilience for regeneration. However, the truth is simple: cartilage doesn't repair itself because you're under 40. Ligaments don't re-knit because you've still got a mortgage to pay and arthritis doesn't hold back because you're "too young" for it.

What youth gives you is not immunity but higher activity levels. That means more stress, more strain and more chance of a small issue being accelerated into a major one. In some ways, waiting in your thirties and forties is more destructive than waiting later in life, because you're still pushing your body hard while the problem brews.

What I See in Clinic

The patterns are almost predictable:
- **The runner with persistent knee pain** who keeps training "through it". By the time they stop, the cartilage is worn and arthritis has started years earlier than it should.

- **The desk worker with a slipped disc** who adapts their posture and ups their medication instead of addressing it properly. Months turn into years and by then nerve damage has taken root.
- **The amateur footballer who tears a ligament** but skips structured rehab. A year later, the knee is unstable, the gait has changed and hip and back pain have joined the party. Worse, the enjoyment of playing has been lost.

None of these people are "old". Yet all of them suffer outcomes made worse by one thing: delay.

The biggest barrier for younger patients isn't the body, it's the brain. They feel they don't have time to be injured - careers are at their peak, families are busy, mortgages need paying. The idea of stepping off the treadmill for surgery or structured rehab feels impossible.

Instead they carry on, not realising that by "saving time" they are spending it in another currency. They spend it in poorer sleep, shorter tempers and missed family moments or in hobbies that become too painful to keep up. By the time they finally seek help, the original window has closed and what could have been corrected with relative ease has hardened into permanent restriction.

What Younger Patients Need to Hear

Here's the truth:
- **You don't get rewarded for ignoring pain.** Endurance doesn't build resilience; it builds damage.

- **Acting early preserves decades.** One decision at 40 can protect your 60s, 70s and beyond.
- **Health is not indulgence.** It's the foundation that makes everything else possible: work, family, sport, travel.

Younger patients are often meticulous about financial investments. They service their cars, insure their homes and top up their pensions. When it comes to their bodies though, they treat repair as optional.

My Quick Guide: When Not to Wait

Your body doesn't hand out medals for "soldiering on". Here's how to know when to stop waiting and act.

 Mild Signals (Don't ignore these. They're the warm-up act for bigger problems.)
- Persistent pain that doesn't settle after rest (48-hour rule – if it's not better get a scan)
- Stiffness in the morning lasting more than 30 minutes.
- Recurring swelling in a joint or limb.
- Breathlessness doing things that used to feel easy (like stairs).
- Fatigue that lingers for weeks, not days.

Translation: This is your body flashing warning lights.

 Moderate Signals (Book the appointment. "Wait and see" is no longer a strategy.)
- Pain that wakes you at night.
- Noticeable loss of movement (can't lift your arm overhead, can't bend your knee fully).

- Numbness, tingling, or weakness in hands or feet.
- Sudden changes in vision or hearing.
- Shortness of breath even at rest.

Translation: This is your boiler leaking and you know you need a plumber.

 Severe Signals (Stop reading. Get help - this is urgent.)
- Chest pain or tightness that doesn't ease quickly.
- Sudden severe headache, slurred speech, or facial droop (possible stroke).
- High fever with confusion or rapid breathing (possible sepsis).
- Rapid, unexplained weight loss.
- Loss of bladder or bowel control with back pain (spinal red flag).

Translation: This is like your house being on fire, you need to call for professionals.

Delay compounds damage, always. What you put off today doesn't just wait patiently, it multiplies. So, ask yourself: what are you ignoring right now? The ache, the swelling, the fatigue you're writing off as "normal"?

Why Monitoring Progress Keeps You From Wasting Months or Years

The Psychological Trap: "I Think It's Better"

One of the most dangerous phrases I hear in clinic is: *"I think it's better."*

What people usually mean is: *"I've stopped noticing it."* Those are not the same thing.

Your brain is extraordinarily clever at adapting to pain and dysfunction. It can dial pain down in the background, reroute your movement patterns and convince you that things are fine. Yet what's really happening is that you've normalised the problem. The biology hasn't changed; your perception has.

I see this every week. A patient says their knee feels "fine" now, yet when we measure, one leg is 25% weaker than the other. Another insists their shoulder "doesn't hurt anymore", but motion analysis shows they've simply stopped reaching overhead, shifting the load onto their spine instead. They've traded pain for restriction and because the brain accepts that trade without question, they call it recovery.

There's also a psychological cost. When people rely on "I think it's better", they're operating without visibility. If it hurts again, they feel blindsided and discouraged, as though the recovery has failed. But if they'd been tracking progress, they'd have seen the plateau, the lag, the warning signs. Data turns frustration into clarity.

Think of it like a bank account: you don't decide you're financially secure because you think you have enough money, you check the numbers. Pain and function are the same, your feelings fluctuate; the numbers tell you the truth.

That's why I tell patients: stop guessing, start measuring. Because "I think it's better" is not a strategy; it's a trap. You need objective data, a photo, video, voice memo (a free and powerful app on your smartphone) or of course MAI-Motion.

The Drift Problem

One of the most common things people say when they finally come to see me is this: *"It all happened suddenly"*. Their back went or a shoulder froze, yet when we look more closely, there has been a steady pattern or erosion of movement.

The trouble is you don't notice this day by day. It's like watching your child grow, if you see them every morning, you don't spot the difference. Then you look back at a photo from last year and realise how much has changed. That's the danger with health, if you're not monitoring, you don't see the drift.

When you don't track progress, you can lose years without even realising it.

You tell yourself:
- "It's not too bad, I'll keep going."
- "I'll check in when it gets worse."
- "I think it's improving…"

Think of it like sat-nav. If you miss the turn and don't check the map, you can happily drive 100 miles in the wrong direction before realising you've wasted half a tank. Progress without monitoring is exactly that.

Biology Needs Feedback Loops

If there's one thing that excites me as a scientist, it's feedback loops. Biology thrives on them. Hormones pulse, the brain responds, organs adjust. Blood sugar goes up, insulin comes in, oxygen dips, you breathe faster. Feedback is what keeps you alive every second of every day.

Now here's the point: if your body already runs on feedback, you need to do the same. Without it, you're breaking the loop. You're asking your biology to do all the sensing while you stay blind.
- **Pain journals:** If you write down how intense pain is each day, you'll see trends. Otherwise, you just "get used to it".

- **Mobility checks:** Can you squat, bend, or stretch to the same point as last month? A centimetre less doesn't feel like much in a day but over a year it can mean real loss of function.
- **Energy logs:** Are you flagging earlier in the day than before? That's not just "getting older". It's a sign of something changing.

We use longitudinal monitoring in medicine all the time: in trials, in elite sport and in rehab. Ordinary people will wing it; they rely on memory and gut feeling, the problem being that memory lies, whereas monitoring doesn't.

Real-Life Example

David, 45, booked in because his right knee *"suddenly started giving way"*. Mechanically, that's my world and he expected a quick scan and perhaps a cortisone injection.

When we took a proper history, the pattern was slow and predictable: he'd stopped hiking a couple of years earlier, gardening had gone the year after and recently he needed his hands to push off a chair. That's not a single event, that's drift.

To separate story from fact, we ran MAI-Motion and this is where things get objective. MAI-Motion captured how his knee moved under everyday load: stride pattern, load distribution, timing, flexion-extension through the gait cycle and how the joint rotated under stress. Not guesswork but accurate numbers.

Pillar 4 - Time: The Missing Variable

What MAI-Motion showed:

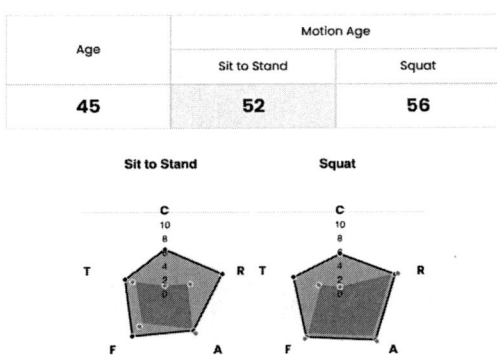

Clear **asymmetry** between limbs: shorter stance time and reduced push-off on the right side.
- A **flattened flexion curve** through loading and mid-stance (he was protecting the joint by not bending it).
- **Altered rotation timing** at the knee during gait, consistent with an irritated meniscus and lax soft tissues.
- Knock-on changes at the hip and trunk from months of compensation.

In plain English: the knee wasn't just painful; it had **reorganised his movement**. That's why it felt "unreliable".

Now the useful bit. We used that MAI-Motion dataset in two ways:
1. **Decision point, rehab first or surgery soon?**
   The motion profile told us there was still capacity to recover if we restored strength and control quickly. We set a **12-week monitored block**: targeted quadriceps

and hip work, balance drills matched to his deficits and gait retraining to reopen the flexion he'd been avoiding.
2. **If he failed rehab, plan a personalised operation, not a generic one.**
   If symptoms persisted or instability remained, those same MAI-Motion curves would be fed into **Twis-TKR** (the knee replacement technique I pioneered) so the implant position and soft-tissue balance could be tailored to David's actual movement pattern, not an average. That's the point of MAI-Motion in Twis-TKR: **customisation from real motion**.

Monitoring progress, not guessing:
We repeated MAI-Motion at 6 and 12 weeks. The aim wasn't a perfect score; it was a **trend**:
- Stance time on the right moved towards symmetry.
- The flexion curve regained shape through loading (he stopped guarding).
- Rotation timing normalised.
- Subjectively, the "giving way" episodes disappeared.

Having measured, we didn't waste six months "hoping". We had a timescale, clear thresholds and a back-up plan. Had those curves stayed flat, we would have escalated promptly and used the same data to individualise a Twis-TKR.

Without MAI-Motion, David's path would have been guesswork, periods of rest, a few random exercises, another flare and eventually a late referral. With MAI-Motion, we had **evidence, timelines and options**. That's how you stop months turning into years.

Pillar 4 - Time: The Missing Variable

How MAI-Motion Can Help You Too

You don't need a dramatic injury for MAI-Motion to be useful. In fact, it is most powerful long before things "go wrong".

Most people live with subtle changes for years: a shorter stride, a joint that avoids load, a side that does a little less work. None of this feels urgent. It just feels like ageing, stiffness or being out of shape. Over time, those small adaptations compound and what began as compensation becomes limitation.

MAI-Motion makes that drift visible.

By analysing how you move under everyday load, it shows where force is being absorbed well and where it is leaking away. It measures symmetry, timing, joint sequencing and how load travels through your body, not in isolation, but as a connected system. This turns vague symptoms into objective information.

For most people, that data answers three critical questions:
1. **Am I adapting or deteriorating?**
   A joint can hurt yet still function well, or feel fine while quietly losing capacity. MAI-Motion distinguishes between protective patterns that can be reversed and changes that are already limiting resilience.
2. **What actually needs attention right now?**
   Instead of generic exercises or blanket advice, the data points to specific deficits: strength, control, timing or coordination. That means less wasted effort and faster progress.

3. **What is my window of opportunity?**
   Time matters. MAI-Motion helps define whether there is still room to rebuild capacity conservatively or whether intervention should be escalated sooner, with a clear plan rather than hope.

The real value is not a single scan but the ability to track change. Repeating MAI-Motion at defined intervals shows whether your system is adapting in the right direction. Improvement becomes measurable. Plateaus become obvious. Decisions stop being delayed by uncertainty.

This is how you prevent drift turning into decline. By measuring movement early, responding precisely and adjusting before months become years.

Monitoring

There's a whole field called longitudinal monitoring, tracking change over time. Medicine uses it all the time in trials. Athletes use it religiously in training.

- Track blood pressure over years and you can predict stroke risk.
- Track bone density and you can prevent fractures.
- Track blood sugar and you can delay diabetes complications.

It's not complicated science; it's just consistency. If you don't monitor, you don't manage.

How Monitoring Turns Guesswork Into Knowledge

The difference between those who hold onto health and those who slide into decline isn't luck. It's whether they notice the changes when they're small enough to do something about.

If you track your:
- **Blood pressure**, you can spot hypertension before it leads to stroke.
- **Bone density**, you can prevent fractures before they happen.
- **Blood sugar**, you can change lifestyle before diabetes complications lock in.
- **Mobility and strength**, you can adapt your exercise before arthritis or frailty take over.
- **Sleep patterns**, you can spot drifting bedtimes, rising night-wakings and shrinking deep sleep long before fatigue, weight gain or cognitive decline become obvious.

The science is simple: what you monitor, you can manage. What you ignore, you lose.

The Exciting Part: Why This Works

The biology behind monitoring is elegant: muscles adapt to use, bones adapt to stress and nerves adapt to demand. Of course adaptation cuts both ways; if you don't challenge a system, it declines.

The beauty of monitoring is that it shows you where the tipping points are. You don't need to wait until your hip has collapsed, or until you can't breathe going up the stairs. Small, measurable changes show you what's coming, that means you can act *before* the damage compounds.

I'll go back to the finance example, you wouldn't check your bank balance once every three years, you'd have no idea what was going in or out. You'd wake up one day and wonder where all the money had gone. That's what people do with their health when they don't monitor it. They wake up one day wondering where their mobility, strength, or energy went. It didn't vanish overnight; they just weren't watching.

Monitoring your time leads to true regeneration.

Real-Life Example

Emma, 28, came in after an ACL reconstruction. The surgery had gone well. What she hadn't realised was that the real work starts afterwards. She had done some rehab, then stopped tracking it. No strength data, no balance data, just the vague sense that "it should be fine by now".

When we tested her, the difference was obvious: her reconstructed leg was still 30% weaker than the other side. That weakness was invisible to her in daily life, but it showed up every time she jogged. Her gait had shifted, her hip was compensating and her cartilage was taking the strain.

This wasn't about effort. She was exercising. The problem was lack of measurement. Without data, you can't see progress. Without progress markers, you can't adjust.

We brought in regular quad strength tests, hop symmetry measures and proprioception drills. Within weeks, Emma could see the graphs change. Her motivation returned, her rehab became specific and the gap began to close.

That's the point: ACL surgery doesn't fail because of the operation. It fails because people miss the rehab window and once that window closes, the risk isn't just another ligament tear, it's a knee that ages ten years faster than it should.

Monitoring Isn't Complicated

People think monitoring means complicated gadgets, but it doesn't. You can download apps, buy wearable tech, or fancy tests but you don't have to. Some of the best monitoring is the simplest:

- Write your pain score (0–10) in a notebook each evening.
- Time how long it takes to climb a flight of stairs once a month.
- Note how many times you wake at night each week.
- Check your blood pressure every few weeks at the pharmacy.
- Download MAI-Motion.

These things take minutes, but over months and years, they add up to knowledge that can save you decades.

Practical Toolkit: How to Monitor Without Obsession

Patients often ask me, "How much should I be measuring?" My answer is enough to see the truth but not so much that you drive yourself mad. Monitoring should empower you, not imprison you.

Here's how I advise doing it:

1. Pick your top 3–5 markers.
Don't measure twenty things and get lost in spreadsheets. Choose what matters to your situation: pain, mobility, energy, sleep, or a relevant lab marker (blood sugar, blood pressure, cholesterol). Think of them as your personal console dials.

2. Be consistent, not constant.
Weekly or monthly is plenty. You don't need to log pain every hour as biology works in trends, it's the slope of the line that matters, not the wiggles in between.

3. Keep it simple.

Use 0–10 pain scores, minutes walked, or the weight you can lift. These are quick to jot down and easy to understand. Don't over-engineer the process; if it takes too long, you won't stick with it.

4. Visual beats memory.

A simple graph, even drawn in a notebook, is worth more than "I think I'm better". The human brain is terrible at recall. Numbers plotted over time show drift and progress in a way memory simply can't.

5. Review but don't obsess.

Data is for decisions, not drama. Look at the pattern once a week or once a month. If the line is trending down, act early, if it's trending up, celebrate and keep going. The point is clarity, not constant checking.

6. Add a function test.

Don't just record feelings, record function. Can you get out of a chair without using your arms or can you walk up a flight of stairs without stopping? These milestones are often more reliable than pain scores.

7. Set checkpoints.

Book in your own 3-month or 6-month reviews, even if it's just with yourself. Ask yourself: Am I moving better or am I stronger? Is my energy higher?" Formal checkpoints prevent drift into years of *I thought it was fine*.

8. Share the data.

Bring your notes or graphs to appointments. Clinicians make better decisions with real numbers, not vague recollections. It turns a ten-minute consultation into a focused plan, not guesswork.

9. Monitor your 5 Star week.

The chart provided helps you to see what's happening as a clear snapshot. You can download a copy from my website or create your own version.

	Number of Drinks	Number of Urinations
Sunday		
Monday		
Tuesday		
Wednesday		
Thursday		
Friday		
Saturday		

Date	Pain (0–10)	Mobility (mins walked / stairs)	Energy (0–10)	Sleep (hrs)	Function Test (e.g. sit-to-stand)	Urine Stars	Notes
Week 1							
Week 2							
Week 3							
Week 4							

How to Value Your Health at Least as Much as Your Possessions

We'll Do It for the Dog

Ask almost any pet owner what they'd do if their dog started limping. The answer is immediate: *"Straight to the vet"*. No hesitation, no debate. They'll pay hundreds or even thousands for scans, surgery and rehab because they can't bear to see their animal in pain.

Yet when their own hip stiffens or their knee locks, those same people shrug. They "carry on", telling themselves it's just age and waiting years before seeking help. It's one of the greatest contradictions in modern healthcare: we treat our pets with urgency and compassion, but we treat our own bodies as if they're expendable.

That difference in attitude isn't trivial. Your dog gets back to chasing a ball whilst you limp after them, losing muscle, twisting your spine until you can no longer walk the dog, by then there is usually no choice but surgery. On top of that, it's harder, riskier and leaves you permanently limited.

Why We Put Ourselves Last

There are cultural, emotional and financial reasons.
- **Cultural Stoicism.** In Britain especially, there's a badge of honour in "not making a fuss".
- **The Illusion of the NHS.** People feel they've already "paid" through National Insurance. That's true in principle but it doesn't guarantee timely care, the gap between expectation and reality is where decline happens. Public funding also creates a sense of security that doesn't reflect the rising personal costs once you fall outside NHS provision, even briefly.
- **Money Mindset.** Spending on possessions feels easier because you can see the return: a new car, a working boiler or a repaired phone. Spending on health feels invisible until you experience what it gives back.
- **Fear and Denial.** If you don't seek help, you don't have to face the diagnosis. Waiting feels like control.

NHS vs Private: The Value Question

This is where the tension hits hardest. Patients often say: *"I've paid into the NHS all my life, why should I pay privately?"*

The NHS is extraordinary, I worked in it for twenty years. It is a global symbol of fairness, and it saves lives every minute of every day. It is also built on triage and life-threatening illness comes first. Quality of life, mobility, independence, chronic pain and functional decline sit lower on the priority list, not because they aren't important, but because the system has to save the dying before it can optimise the living.

Pillar 4 - Time: The Missing Variable

Orthopaedics is one of the clearest examples. A damaged hip or knee rarely kills you, so it moves down the queue. This happens in hospitals as well as on waiting lists, if an urgent surgery needs an operating theatre, then there is a good chance that a 'non-urgent' surgery will get bumped. The person whose operation is cancelled may have already been waiting twelve months but that won't be seen by the person making the call to save a life.

Private care isn't a rejection of the NHS, it's a recognition of what time does to the body. A knee replaced six weeks after diagnosis behaves very differently to a knee replaced after two years of pain, altered gait and muscle loss. The surgeon and the procedure may be the same, yet the eventual recovery curve is completely different.

Here's the cost people don't factor in: every month spent unable to walk, work or live normally is a month of life permanently removed from circulation. The NHS pays the price too, delayed intervention leads to longer surgery time, slower recovery, more complications and more long-term demand on the system.

The question isn't "NHS or private?" it should be "What is the cost of waiting?"

Real-Life Example

Carol was 80 when I met her. She'd spent most of her life in hospitality, running her own self-catering apartments. That meant decades of heavy work: lifting mattresses, changing bedding, wallpapering, decorating, scrubbing and hauling. It was a career that required strength but also one that slowly took its toll on her shoulders.

Her left shoulder had been replaced on the NHS some years earlier. The result was, in her own words, a disaster. The implant damaged nerves, her elbow stuck out "like a teapot", and she couldn't lift her arm above her head. She told the story with humour but behind it was the reality: pain, loss of function and a deep erosion of trust.

Then, when her right shoulder began to fail, Carol hesitated. She was in severe pain, struggling with the simplest tasks but the memory of her first operation hung over her like a shadow. Every time the subject came up, she shook her head: *"Never again"*.

Her family suggested she consider private care. Carol's first response was one I hear often: *"I've paid into the NHS all my life. Why should I spend money on something I've already funded?"* She saw private surgery not as investment but as betrayal. Paying felt like undermining a system she believed in and had contributed to faithfully.

The second barrier was fear. If her left shoulder had gone so wrong, why would the right one be any better? What if she spent a large sum, savings carefully built over a lifetime, only to be left in the same pain, or worse? To her, the risk felt unbearable.

So, Carol waited. She endured the pain, adapted her movements and told herself she could live with it. As months passed though, the pain grew and her independence shrank. Sleep became fractured, daily tasks became ordeals and she found herself exhausted simply from the effort of avoiding certain movements. What had once been stubborn loyalty to the NHS became quiet suffering.

Finally, she reached a breaking point and she realised she couldn't go on. The NHS list stretched endlessly into the distance and her pain was now unmanageable. With her family's encouragement, she decided, reluctantly, to go private.

The difference was like night and day. From the first consultation, she was listened to, given time and offered clear explanations. On the day of surgery, she was cared for with dignity, the operation itself was smooth, without complication and after her recovery, for the first time in years, Carol found she could raise her right arm higher than her left.

The irony wasn't lost on her. The operation she had resisted most fiercely, the one she feared would waste her savings and repeat the disaster of her past, turned out to restore her more function and comfort than the "free" operation that had failed her.

Carol's story highlights three realities patients often wrestle with:
- **Affordability** and feeling they have "already paid" can make people delay treatment they desperately need.
- **Fear of past experiences** can paralyse decision-making.
- **The cost of waiting,** in pain, in lost independence, in quality of life, is always higher than the cost of timely action.

When we talked afterwards, she admitted something quietly: *"I should have done it sooner"*. That single sentence is one I've heard countless times.

The truth is, Carol wasn't wrong to value the NHS. None of us should take it for granted but valuing the NHS and valuing yourself are not the same thing. One does not cancel out the other. Her outcome proved that timely investment in her own health was not indulgence, rather it was wisdom, that returned her movement, her comfort and her confidence in her final years of life.

The Economics of Health vs Possessions

Many people wouldn't think twice about spending £20,000 on a car. They'll finance it, stretch their budget, make it work, yet the idea of spending £20,000 on a hip replacement feels extravagant.

Ask yourself – what is a car without the ability to drive it or what's a dream holiday if you can't walk to the plane? What's the point of savings if you can't live well enough to enjoy them?

Health is the platform that makes every possession usable. Lose health and possessions become meaningless.

The Biology of Waiting

When you delay, it's not that the body is doing nothing. It's busy, just not in ways you want.

A 40-year-old who acts early on a meniscus tear may get it repaired and return to sport. The same 40-year-old who waits until 50 may face a joint replacement and permanent limitations. The biology is the same, the difference is time.

Health as an Asset

Here's the reframe I give patients: your health is your greatest asset. Not in sentimental terms but in economic reality. It underpins everything else: work, family, travel, independence.

You track your finances, you maintain your tech and you monitor your family – at what point do you add your wellbeing to the unconscious monitoring you're doing of everything else?

Practical Toolkit:
The Health Value Audit

Fill this in honestly. It will show you in black and white whether you're valuing your health or undervaluing it compared to everything else in life.

1. Would You Do It for Your Pet?
- How much do you spend each month on pet insurance? £_____
- What do you currently spend on private medical insurance? £_____

Gap: _____

2. The Real Cost of Waiting
- How many months/years have you already lost to pain? _____
- What can't you currently do (e.g. walk far, sleep well, travel, play with grandchildren)?

Multiply: Lost months × activities missed = The true cost of waiting.

3. Expense vs Investment
- Surgery/rehab cost: £_____
- Expected benefit (years of function/independence gained): _____ years
- Cost ÷ Years gained = £_____ per year of better life.

(Compare: a new car depreciates faster than that.)

4. Health as Insurance
Tick what you currently insure:
- ☐ Car   (£_____/year)
- ☐ House (£_____/year)
- ☐ Phone (£_____/year)

Now write:
- My body is worth: £_____ per year.
- Am I investing that? Yes ☐ No ☐

5. Loyalty Check
- Have you told yourself, "I've paid into the NHS all my life"? Yes ☐ No ☐
- If yes, ask: would freeing up NHS time by going private actually help others in greater need? Write your answer:

_____

_____

6. The Five-Year Question

- If I act now, in five years I will:

_____

- If I delay, in five years I will:

_____

Decision: Act Now ☐   Delay ☐

Were you completely honest and how did it make you feel?

Valuing your health at least as much as your possessions isn't indulgence. It's the most rational, compassionate decision you can make. Because the truth is simple: you can replace a car or a phone. But you cannot replace the years lost to pain.

Ageing Better: Why Mindset Matters as Much as Medicine

If you lined up photos of forty-year-olds today with forty-year-olds from the 1970s, you'd swear they were a different generation. Back then, forty often looked like sixty: thicker waists, greyer hair, clothes that screamed "middle-aged" the moment you put them on. Fast forward to now and forty looks leaner, sharper and frankly a lot more fun. People in their sixties are running marathons, starting new businesses and wearing trainers instead of orthopaedic shoes (although with good arch support).

This isn't just vanity, something deeper is going on. We're *acting younger* and *feeling younger* and that mindset isn't just cosmetic, it genuinely changes the way the body regenerates.

Biology Listens to Belief

One of the most fascinating findings in modern ageing science is that your biology doesn't just respond to pills, diet, or exercise, it responds to belief. If you feel younger than your chronological age, research shows you're more likely to have lower inflammation, stronger immunity and better heart health. You literally live longer.

I see this in clinic every week, patients who tell me, "I still feel thirty inside", often move better, recover faster and engage with rehab like they're training for a personal best. Patients who tell me, "Well, I'm just old now", slump into the chair before we've even started. Same age yet different mindset and biology respond accordingly.

This is mental behaviour. Feel younger and you *act* younger. You keep walking, you stretch, you eat well, you try and your cells reward you for it. Feel older and you withdraw; you stop doing things and your cells respond to that too.

Ancient Wisdom Got There First

Now here's something cool. Modern science is proving what ancient traditions were saying thousands of years ago.
- **Greek philosophy**: The Greeks talked about *eukrasia*: balance of the humours. They trained both body and mind because they believed decline came from imbalance, not just age itself. If you kept balance, you extended vitality. That's regeneration thinking, 2,000 years ago.
- **Chinese medicine**: Traditional Chinese medicine saw ageing as a decline in *qi* (vital energy) and blood flow. The answer wasn't denial but daily correction. Herbs, tai chi, acupuncture and food choices were all designed to keep the system fluid and resilient. They assumed you'd age but they assumed you could slow it, bend it and regenerate within it.

- **Ayurveda**: In India, Ayurveda mapped human life into stages. The later years weren't written off, they were reframed: lighter food, more meditation, oil massage and herbal tonics. The point was to extend clarity and movement as long as possible, not to collapse into decline.

What strikes me is this: none of these traditions treated ageing as an enemy. They treated it as a rhythm to be respected. You don't fight time; you dance with it.

Modern Science is Catching Up

Here's the beautiful part. We now have the data to show they were right.
- Movement done daily and consistently rather than dramatically, alters inflammatory markers and slows cellular ageing.
- Meditation and breathwork, once shrugged off as fringe practices, are now shown to reduce cortisol, regulate heart rhythms and improve immunity.
- Balanced diets, with the right mix of protein, healthy fats and plant-supported nutrients, reduce oxidative stress and feed regeneration at the cellular level. Too much of one thing, whether meat or plants, tips you off balance. The trick is variety, not extremism.

Every time a study comes out, I find myself smiling, because we're rediscovering what the ancients already intuited. They didn't have MRIs or CRP blood tests, but they saw the outcomes.

External Youth vs Internal Truth

Of course, modern life has also given us cheats. Hair dye, fillers, Botox, fashion: they all help us look younger and there's nothing wrong with that. Here's the key though, looking younger is only powerful if it feeds into *acting younger*. The danger is when the mirror fools you into complacency.

If you feel good, brilliant, now use that energy to keep moving, keep strengthening, keep regenerating. If you rely only on the cosmetic, you miss the point.

Time as an Ally, Not an Enemy

The most important reframe is this: time doesn't have to be adversary. Yes, delay compounds damage when you ignore it, but time also compounds benefits when you act.

Start strength training at forty and you carry those benefits into your fifties, sixties, seventies. Sort your sleep at fifty and you regulate hormones, energy and recovery for decades. Intervene on a joint before collapse and you may never need a replacement.

This is the regenerative mindset: time multiplies *whatever* you feed it. If you give it neglect, it multiplies decline, yet if you give it care, it multiplies strength.

Pulling It Together: Ancient Wisdom, Modern Tools

If you want to know where regeneration really happens, it's not in choosing one camp, ancient or modern, it's in combining them.

- **Respect the clock.** You can't cheat time. Joints, tendons and cartilage all carry your age in their fibres. Acknowledging that doesn't mean surrender, it means working *with* the biology of time, not pretending it isn't there.
- **Mindset as biology.** This isn't mild psychology. Believing you're younger keeps you active and activity keeps your mitochondria, muscles and hormones tuned. Your body literally listens to your attitude.
- **Ancient daily rituals.** Whether it's tai chi, yoga, or Ayurveda's insistence on regularity, the ancients understood that small daily rhythms compound over decades. They weren't being mystical; they were being practical about slowing wear and tear. Find a local club while you're working on your body and you'll also meet likeminded people, which is also good for your mental health.
- **Modern interventions.** Here's where we have the edge. We can scan cartilage before it fails, replace joints with precision implants, use MAI-Motion to analyse movement in a way Hippocrates would have been amazed by. The ancients gave us rhythm; modern medicine gives us repair. Together, they're far stronger than either alone.

The point is this: you don't have to choose between old and new. Regeneration happens when you respect the lessons of both.

We live in an extraordinary era. We can look younger, feel younger and with the right habits and interventions, regenerate younger. Time will keep marching on but whether it marches over you, or marches with you, depends on how you respond.

How Science Is Changing the Future of Time

For centuries, time was a tyrant. It marched in one direction, took what it wanted and never gave anything back. Wrinkles deepened, joints wore thin, muscles faded, memories slipped. Medicine could patch, soothe, or replace but never rewind.

That's the old story.

The new story is that science is starting to make time feel less like a straight line and more like something we can bend, stretch and even recycle. We're not talking about science fiction but real tools that are beginning to change what "ageing" and "regeneration" mean.

From Countdown to Clock Management

As I've already said, your biology is a set of clocks. For most of history, they ticked down without pause. Bone density clock, muscle mass clock, hormone clock, brain plasticity clock, all running out at their own pace.

The exciting shift in science is that we're not just watching these clocks anymore, we're learning how to **intervene in them**.

- **Pause some clocks.**
  Take muscle loss, for example. After about 40, muscle mass naturally starts to decline. Left unchecked, this leads to frailty, slower recovery from injury and higher risk of falls. Targeted resistance training, even twice a week, slows this dramatically. Add in nutritional support and suddenly the "inevitable" isn't so inevitable. On the molecular level, researchers are exploring how the mTOR pathway (one of the body's main growth and repair switches) can be modulated to keep muscle and cell repair more active for longer. Pausing doesn't mean stopping forever, it means holding onto strength and resilience for years beyond what biology once allowed.
- **Reset others.**
  Here's where it gets futuristic. Epigenetics, the software that tells your DNA what to do, doesn't just age in one direction. Early studies suggest it can be **rewound**. That means a cell that looks and behaves like a "60-year-old" can, under the right conditions, be rolled back to act like a "30-year-old". We're not talking science fiction: reprogramming factors have already shown this in labs. Imagine what that means for tissues like cartilage, skin, or even organs. It's not about chasing immortality; it's about restoring lost function, re-opening repair windows that biology used to close.
- **Synchronise them.**
  What comes next isn't just about slowing individual processes; it's about synchronising them.

Circadian biology shows that when the clocks in your brain, muscles, liver and immune system run together, repair is amplified. Hormones are released when tissues are primed to respond, inflammation switches off at the right moment, and recovery becomes faster and more complete. This is where science is heading: therapies that bring every clock into alignment so the whole system regenerates at its best.

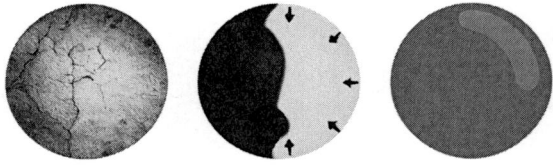

In other words, time is becoming something we manage, not just endure.

Extending Repair Windows

One of the most exciting questions in regenerative science is this: what if the windows we thought were closed could be reopened? Traditionally, biology gives you a one-time shot, heal now, or live with the consequences. Now new science is showing that might not always be true.

- **Gene editing** is already proving we can correct inherited errors long after birth. What used to be written in stone is now more like a draft we can edit.
- **Cellular reprogramming** goes further. By rewinding the epigenetic clock, we may be able to take tissues that have stiffened, scarred, or aged and restore them to a more youthful, regenerative state.

- **Bioengineered scaffolds** are being designed as physical platforms for repair. In the past, a damaged joint or organ that scarred over was written off as "too late". Now, we're learning how to give cells a new structure to grow into, effectively telling biology to "start again".

This is the frontier: shifting from a model where time shuts the door, to one where we learn how to prise it open again. Repair that doesn't expire when the dates say it should.

Borrowing From the Future

Another way to think about it: medicine is learning to **borrow time from the future and bring it forward**.
- Banking stem cells while you're young to use them decades later.
- Freezing eggs or sperm to extend fertility years beyond biology's old limits.
- Collecting personal movement data now (MAI-Motion systems) so your "normal" gait can be restored if you ever need surgery.

Cryogenics is the extreme end of this idea; the hope that you can literally press pause on your whole body and wake up in a future where regeneration is limitless. Most of us won't sign up for liquid nitrogen storage but the principle is already alive in everyday medicine: *preserve now, use later.*

Time as a Regenerative Resource

The most radical change in thinking is this: time itself is becoming a resource we can shape.

- **Slowing time.** Longevity research isn't about making people live forever; it's about extending *healthspan*: the years when your body regenerates effectively. Drugs targeting pathways like mTOR and sirtuins are being tested not to add decades of decline but to stretch the period of strength, repair and resilience. It's not "older for longer" it's "younger for longer".
- **Bending time.** For the first time, we can measure biological age separately from the number on your passport. AI-driven biological age clocks analyse DNA methylation, protein profiles, even movement patterns and can tell you if your cells are ageing faster or slower than your lifespan suggests. That means time is no longer just chronological, it's biological and if it's measurable, it's adjustable.
- **Reversing time.** The most audacious work is in epigenetic reprogramming and senolytics. Early trials suggest we can clear out damaged, senescent cells, the "zombie cells" that clog up tissues and even roll them back to a younger state. Lab mice have had their vision restored and muscle function renewed by tweaking these switches. It's not mythology or alchemy; it's measured in labs today.

For regeneration, this is seismic. It means you're no longer entirely at the mercy of your internal logbook. The conversation is shifting from "how long do you have left?" to "how well are your cells using the time you've got?" What sounds like science fiction is science, right now, nudging time from a fixed force into a therapeutic tool.

Ancient Dreams, Modern Tools

The longing to stop time isn't a modern obsession. It has always been there, stitched into human history. Every culture has tried to outsmart the clock.

The alchemists spent centuries chasing the elixir of life, convinced that somewhere in the bubbling crucibles lay a way to outwit ageing. For the Taoists, immortality wasn't magic but balance, movement, breath, ritual, all designed to keep the body in rhythm with nature. The Egyptians, masters of preservation, embalmed their dead in the hope that eternal youth might be waiting on the other side.

There's also myth and stories. The Fountain of Youth, promised by explorers who thought water itself could rinse away the years. The Greek gods kept forever young on ambrosia and later, literature gave us Oscar Wilde's The Picture of Dorian Gray, a man who never aged while his portrait bore the marks of time and corruption. That book still grips us because it touches the raw truth: ageing feels like betrayal.

What links all of these? The refusal to accept that biology has hard deadlines. Whether through potions, embalming, or fantasy, people have always tried to stretch time, pause it, or reverse it.

What's different now is that for the first time, the tools are real. We don't have elixirs, but we do have molecules like rapamycin and senolytics, being tested to extend "healthspan" by clearing damaged cells. We don't embalm bodies, but we do use cryogenics, the modern echo of ancient preservation, keeping the possibility of future revival alive in tanks of liquid nitrogen. We don't consult prophets, but we do consult AI-driven biological clocks that tell us if our cells are ageing faster or slower than our birthdays say. Where Dorian Gray had a painting, we now have epigenetic reprogramming: a way of winding tissues back towards a younger state in the lab.

The dream hasn't changed. People want to be younger for longer. What's changed is that we've shifted from myth to measurable science. The ancients relied on ritual, symbol and hope. We now have MRI scans, gene editing, stem cells and motion analysis. Their vision was the same as ours, to stretch regeneration into years when biology normally says "enough".

The fantasy of eternal youth may always stay just out of reach, but the science of extended regeneration is moving from fiction to fact. The tools are finally catching up with the dream.
The dream hasn't changed: people want to be younger for longer. The tools finally have.

The Practical Takeaway

So, what does this mean for you, right now? It means that regeneration is no longer just about patching the present. It's about positioning yourself for the future:
1. **Act early.** Every year that you bank healthy habits, you extend your repair window.
2. **Think long-term.** Store data, monitor progress and keep options open for future therapies.

3. **Stay open.** What seems experimental today may be mainstream in 10 years. Patients who are prepared can step straight in when the science is ready.
4. **Value your time.** Don't waste the regenerative years you already have waiting for the "perfect" future treatment. Use what works now, while keeping an eye on what's next.

Now the story of time in medicine is changing, it's no longer just a countdown. It's becoming a collaboration and what's next for regeneration isn't about defying time completely, it's about making time work for you, instead of against you.

Why I engineered the Regen PhD Pod

After years in theatres and clinics, I knew patients didn't just want surgery, they wanted answers. They wanted precision, predictability and regeneration, not replacement. The Pod grew out of a single question: what happens if you combine the right forms of energy and signal delivery, hold them steady long enough for biology to respond and measure it in real time?

The result is technology designed to work with the body's timing and physiology rather than against it: heat to encourage relaxation and healthy blood flow; light to increase cellular energy; vibration to ease tight tissue without triggering flare-ups; magnetic fields that help regulate electrical behaviour in the body; and targeted scents selected for specific effects such as focus, calm, or recovery.

Each element timed, tuned and coordinated by an adaptive brain.

It's about bringing the whole system into alignment, so repair becomes reliable. The Pod exists to put force and timing back under your control, because that's when regeneration stops being chance and starts becoming predictable.

The Pod is my way of working with time, not against it. It turns time from something that slips away into something you can finally use, deliberately, for regeneration.

When your timing aligns with nature's, the body rewards you and the pod can help you to reset.

Rhythm is what keeps you young, not just by age but by function. It is how you stop the clock without trying to fight it.

But recovery is only half the story. If you want regeneration, you have to give the body a reason to adapt in the first place.

Chapter Summary

Time is the factor that decides whether regeneration happens cleanly or collapses into compensation, scar tissue and decline. Physics explains structure, chemistry explains inputs, biology explains living systems, but time is the frame that determines whether any of it works.

Time is not neutral. In the body, delay compounds. Small problems do not sit still while someone waits, they reorganise movement, deepen inflammation, train pain pathways, and narrow future options.

The section centres on a blunt biological truth: healing runs on deadlines. Bones, ligaments, nerves and muscles all follow phased repair cycles with critical windows. Act inside the window and tissue can restore strength and function. Miss it and repair becomes messier: fibres tangle into scar tissue, joints stiffen, movement strategies harden, and the nervous system can learn pain. The longer the delay, the more the body adapts around the problem, until one issue becomes several.

Time is framed as a currency more expensive than money, because it cannot be recovered. This pillar challenges the cultural habit of waiting it out, especially the British reflex to soldier on, and contrasts it with elite sport and good medicine, where timing is treated as essential. It also draws a clear parallel with how quickly people act to protect possessions, pets or property, while tolerating years of physical warning lights.

A major theme is feedback. Monitoring prevents drift and replaces guesswork with evidence. The text introduces longitudinal monitoring as the simple discipline that keeps small changes visible before they become irreversible. Examples show how objective measurement, including MAI-Motion, can turn vague symptoms into measurable patterns, set time-limited rehab blocks, guide decision points, and escalate early when thresholds are not improving. The point is not perfect numbers but trends, timelines and options.

The pillar widens beyond joints to highlight silent countdowns in major systems, where delay changes outcomes: stroke and heart attack, liver and kidney decline, lung damage, diabetes complications, vision loss from glaucoma or macular degeneration, and the high stakes of cancer and sepsis. Age is presented as the universal multiplier: the same delay costs more later because repair capacity narrows and recovery budgets shrink.

The practical output is structured around acting early, respecting warning signs, protecting movement, fuelling repair, intervening before chronic pain wiring, and recognising that ageing demands faster decisions, not slower ones.

The overall message is simple: time will compound whatever it is fed. Neglect multiplies decline, but timely action and measurement multiply recovery and preserve future function.

Practical Toolkit: Working With Time

Purpose:
To stop repair windows being wasted through delay, guessing or passive waiting.

Question	Your Answer
Have my symptoms lasted longer than 10–14 days?	Yes ☐ No ☐
Have I clearly identified when this problem started?	Yes ☐ No ☐
Am I inside a likely repair window (early, changeable stage)?	Yes ☐ Unsure ☐
Have I set a defined action period (6–12 weeks)?	Yes ☐ No ☐
Have I written down what I am doing during this period?	Yes ☐ No ☐
Am I measuring at least one functional marker (not just pain)?	Yes ☐ No ☐
Do I have a review date booked at the end of the block?	Yes ☐ No ☐
Do I know what action I will take if there is no improvement?	Yes ☐ No ☐

Functional Markers (tick what applies)

Marker	Tracking Method
☐ Walking tolerance	Minutes / distance
☐ Sit-to-stand ease	Arms needed? Yes ☐ No ☐
☐ Stair tolerance	Stops required? Yes ☐ No ☐
☐ Joint confidence	Stable ☐ Unreliable ☐
☐ Sleep quality	Hours / interruptions
☐ Energy levels	Morning ☐ Afternoon ☐
☐ Strength symmetry	Left ☐ Right ☐
☐ Movement quality	Video / MAI-Motion

Decision Checkpoint

Outcome	Action
☐ Clear improvement	Continue current plan
☐ Partial improvement	Adjust load / strategy
☐ No improvement	Escalate assessment
☐ Deterioration	Stop and reassess immediately

Time Rule

If you have not defined the window, measured progress and set a review point, you are not managing time. Time is managing you.

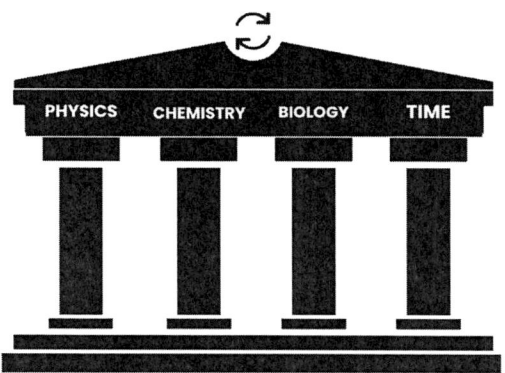

Habits

> *"Regeneration can come only through a change of heart in the individual."*
> *Henry Williamson*

The Crown: The Habits of Regeneration

As you can see, regeneration isn't hard – but it's not exactly easy either. It requires you to consider your entire body, all of the time. That's something we've largely forgotten how to do. Most of us respond only to symptoms; the alarms our bodies sound. Our stomach rumble's and so, we eat. Have a dry mouth, we drink. A headache, let's take a painkiller or an ache, we'll stretch. However, those reactions are just fire-fighting and we don't even link the reactions and consider that the headache and dry mouth are possibly both signs that we haven't drank enough. These signs are maintenance at best.

Chronic pain doesn't behave like ordinary aches because it doesn't ease with a stretch or disappear after a decent night's sleep, it threads itself through how you move, think, and plan the day. When pain dictates the pace, motivation won't carry you. You need systems that hold you up on the days when getting out of bed is a battle and the hours ahead feel too much to take in. For anyone living with ongoing pain, regeneration isn't a luxury or an add-on, it can become the structure that makes the day possible.

Most people still approach health reactively. We sit through the annual MOT, hear the familiar advice about losing a little weight or keeping an eye on cholesterol, nod along, and genuinely intend to do better. Then real life steps in. By the time the appointment ends, the inbox is overflowing, the day has its own demands, and those good intentions begin to slip. At the next supermarket shop, convenience wins, and the plan to "start fresh" dissolves under the pressure of getting through another week.

Overwork is one of the most common reasons people abandon good intentions. It's not idleness; it's the culture we live in. Work emails that don't stop, deadlines piling up and the pressure to perform convince us that health can wait. We've made ourselves contactable 24/7 – gone are the days of clocking off at 4pm on a Friday and forgetting work until 8am Monday morning. Overwork is one of the fastest routes to chronic pain, fatigue and decline. The body can carry that load for a while, then it shows you the cost: stiff shoulders, a sore back and unrefreshing sleep. These aren't isolated symptoms; they are your workload expressed through tissue.

Time – everyone wants more of it – whether it's an extra ten minutes in bed or an extra week off to recover. But time is finite and in some ways, it's the biggest nemesis of regeneration, simply because we've been conditioned to waste it. We take shortcuts with our health because the day's already full. Many patients I've seen would rather have surgery than spend 30 minutes a day stretching, exercising, or simply giving their body what it needs. Not because they're lazy, but because they don't believe they have the time to take care of themselves.

Let me ask you something: are you really not worth half an hour a day? You give your energy to everyone else – to work, to family, to obligation. Would you rather put your body through something invasive and painful, than give yourself care, attention and recovery?

If I asked you outright, you'd probably say, *"Of course not, Paul. I'm worth more than that."* However, the reality is, time and time again, people choose the quicker fix. They rush recovery to get back to work, push through injury to avoid missing out and let the modern world decide what their body needs – therein lies the problem.

> *"A man with health has many dreams. A man without it has only one."* –Hippocrates

Hippocrates wasn't alone. Galen, the great Roman physician, taught that balance was the foundation of health, balance of work and rest, heat and cold, effort and recovery. Ancient Chinese and Ayurvedic traditions said the same: when life falls out of rhythm, illness follows. Modern neuroscience has proved them right. Habits are the rhythms of today, the small, repeated patterns that either keep you in balance or drive you out of it. Ignore them and your body drifts into decline but if you honour them you build resilience. What they called balance we now measure in biomarkers and sleep data. Same principle, new tools.

Now, I'd love to say my engineering skills have led me to invent a magic wand that will keep you young, fit and thriving forever. Maybe one day I'll get there but for now, I can only work with the science, technology and expertise available – and with those, I've created a new way forward.

You've already seen how each pillar feeds into the Pod and why the systems work the way they do. What follows isn't a reveal, it's the next step: how to use these ideas with purpose. How to take what you now understand about force, rhythm, load, energy and biology and turn it into something you can actually live with. The Pod, the tools and the daily practices are here to support that, not as theory, but as a workable framework for real lives and real constraints.

Although before we go further, let me be real with you.

People often ask me, *"How do I actually do this? How do I take all this science, this philosophy and apply it to real life without feeling overwhelmed or falling off after a week?"'*

The truth is it starts with routine.

It's not about reading a book and suddenly doing A, B, C, D, E. It's not even about jumping straight into a big life overhaul. It's about building something succinct, something that fits into your life. If this feels familiar, that's intentional. It echoes the Biological, Boring and Brilliant approach we laid out earlier; the small steady things that actually work.

Now, I could say, "Come and join my network and we'll prescribe what you need to do every day. We'll tell you what principles to follow and how." That would feel too pushy and that's not what I'm trying to do here.

The point is this: you set the routine, decide what regeneration looks like for you and build it into your life in a way that's realistic, repeatable and rooted in what matters most.

Consistency beats intensity. Science beats hacks.

Your routine is where regeneration starts.

A Brief History of Habits

Before we get deep into systems and triggers, it's worth asking: what exactly is a habit and where does the idea come from?

The word itself comes from the Latin *habitus*, which literally meant your state, condition, or even the clothes you wore. In other words, a habit was something you "put on". Over time, the meaning shifted from what you wore on the outside to what you repeated on the inside: the actions and behaviours that shape who you are.

The earliest serious writing about habits goes back to Aristotle in the 4th century BCE. In his *Nicomachean Ethics*, he said something that's still quoted today:

> *"We are what we repeatedly do.*
> *Excellence, then, is not an act but a habit."*

He understood that you don't wake up excellent, you get there through repetition, through embedding good practices until they become second nature.

Fast forward to the 13th century and Thomas Aquinas picked this up, saying that habits weren't just actions but "stable qualities". In other words, the more often you repeat something, the more it becomes part of your character, either in a positive or negative direction.

By the 17th and 18th centuries, thinkers like John Locke were talking about habits in education. He believed the repeated actions we experience as children build the foundations of our thinking and behaviour for the rest of our lives.

But it was in the 19th century that William James, the American philosopher and psychologist, gave us one of the most modern descriptions. He called habit:

> *"The enormous flywheel of society, its most precious conservative agent."*

He meant that habits are what keep us steady. They stop us from having to think through every tiny detail, freeing up mental energy for bigger challenges. He also said that by repeating small actions, we lay down tracks in the brain, automatic pathways that make the behaviour easier each time we do it.

Neuroscience now backs him up. We know that habits are essentially neural shortcuts - repeat an action enough and the brain wires it in, making it more efficient and less effortful. That's why you don't have to "decide" to brush your teeth or tie your shoes every day. It's automatic. It's also why bad habits are so hard to break as they're not just behaviours; they're well-trodden brain pathways.

I know that when I talk about building habits for regeneration, I'm standing on the shoulders of some big names. From Aristotle to James to modern neuroscience, the principle hasn't changed: what you repeat, you become. The only question is whether the habits you've built are serving you or sabotaging you.

Regeneration Is A Habit

If you've read this far, then chances are you're already beginning to think differently about your body, your environment and the way you treat time. But knowledge isn't change – habit is.

This chapter is about how we *apply* everything we've covered so far and keep applying it – not perfectly but persistently. What we're building here is an *unbreakable habit*.

To build a habit, you have to plan for it. You have to build it in. Otherwise, you'll never stick to it.

It takes six days to start a habit. Not six weeks or six months – six days. If you can do something for six days in a row, you've cracked the start. That's the ignition.

After that, you need six weeks for it to settle in and become part of how you live. That's the window where behaviour shifts from effort to instinct, from conscious choice to something your body expects. Six days to begin, six weeks to embed.

Even after six weeks, life happens. You might fall off the wagon. That's fine. It's expected.

Psychologists have been saying the same thing for centuries and modern behavioural science agrees. Carol Dweck's work on growth mindset shows that failure isn't a dead end; it's data. James Clear reminds us with his simple rule: never miss twice. Missing once is human, missing twice is the start of a new habit, usually the wrong kind. That's why the six-day, six-week, six-month framework works: it gives you multiple chances to keep the wheel turning.

I'm recommending setting a reminder in your diary, six months from when you started reading and began your new habit. That's your checkpoint. When that day arrives, revisit this book, not necessarily to re-read the whole thing but just to open a page and to re-engage.

Here's the thing: you'll see it differently and likely it'll hit in a different way. Like a film you rewatch a year later and notice something new. You've changed, your situation has changed and most importantly, what you need has changed.

That's how real learning works. It's layered; it's not about cramming everything in at once, it's about repetition and timing.

You don't need to implement all 20 tips from the physics chapter or to become a regeneration monk overnight.

You just need to pick *one thing*. The lowest hanging fruit. The easiest win.

Do that one thing – every day – for six days.

Then keep going for six weeks, that's your foundation.

Check back in six months. Reset. Pick something new. Build again.

That's the start of regeneration. It's not an event; it's a practice. Here's something most people miss: your priorities change. Right now, you might be focused on movement and pain. Later, the priority might be recovery, hormones or energy. Regeneration evolves with you. It isn't about stockpiling tips; it's about using the right principles at the right moment and sticking with them long enough for them to work.

This matters even more if you live with chronic pain. Pain consumes focus and energy, on good days, you may feel capable of everything, on bad days, nothing. That's why the six-day, six-week, six-month rhythm works so well with accrued changes: it removes the need to "feel like it". Pain or no pain, you know what the next step is. Small, consistent actions accumulate even when the pace is slow.

It's like I always say: you don't need to read ten different self-help books. Read one good book – and actually put it into practice. That's where the change happens.

Your wins come from repetition, not reinvention.

Once you get the rhythm of it – the groove – it becomes effortless, not because it's easy but because you're no longer fighting it.

You've designed your day around your health.

You've designed your life around your longevity.

That is the only shortcut that works.

Designing for Success

Let's talk about the *how*.

At this point, we've looked at the why, the when and the what. However, none of it matters if you haven't created the environment that makes it easier to succeed than to fail. That's where real change happens, when you design for success.

People often think success is about willpower. They imagine it's about grit, discipline and "pushing through" but that's a myth. Willpower runs out. Even the strongest person eventually breaks when their environment is set up to work against them. That's why crash diets fail, why unused gym memberships pile up and why people read self-help books without ever applying them. The system was broken before they began.

So how do you change the system? You start by building your day around your biology, not the other way around. Instead of forcing your body to fit into the chaos of modern life, you arrange modern life to serve your biology.

Environment Always Wins

One of the most powerful things I've learned, both as a surgeon and as a regeneration specialist, is that your environment always wins. It doesn't matter how disciplined you are, if your surroundings are working against you, you will eventually revert back to comfort, to convenience, to the path of least resistance.

- If your fridge is full of fizzy drinks and ready meals, willpower won't save you.
- If your trainers are buried at the back of the cupboard, the odds of you going out for a walk drop.
- If your workspace is a jumble of distractions, don't expect focus to magically appear.

That's why your first job is simple: remove friction.

Workplaces are designed to reward burnout. Long hours are praised, skipping lunch is normal and rest is treated as weakness. If you design your environment to overwork, your body will break down. The fix is to flip the script: treat recovery as a meeting. Block out time for breaks in the same way you block out time for calls. Guard them fiercely because if you don't, overwork will design your body for failure.

Make Good Choices Easy

Designing for success means making it easy to do the right thing and slightly harder to do the wrong thing. Small tweaks make a big impact.

- Leave your water bottle out where you can see it.
- Place your walking shoes by the door.
- Put a post-it on your kettle to stretch while it boils.

- Place a piece of fruit next to your coffee mug.
- Charge your phone outside the bedroom so you don't scroll at midnight.

These aren't hacks, they're design choices. They reduce the friction of doing the bad thing and increase the friction of doing the good thing. *"Oh but Prof, I use my phone as my alarm clock,"* you say: buy a cheap digital alarm that won't keep you doomscrolling when you could be sleeping or set a limit on the time you allow yourself to be on social channels.

We like to imagine that success is the result of big dramatic gestures. In truth, success is usually the by-product of design. Make the helpful thing obvious, easy and attractive and make the unhelpful thing less convenient, less visible, less tempting.

Triggers: The Real Drivers of Habit

Even though you can't always control your workload, your kids, your partner, or your dog, you *can* control triggers and triggers matter. Most of what we do each day is cued by triggers we don't even notice.

For regeneration, I teach people to look at four kinds of triggers:
1. **Visual** - what you see around you.
    - Vitamins by the toothbrush.
    - A yoga mat in the lounge.
    - Trainers in the hallway, not hidden in a bag.
2. **Auditory** - what you hear.
    - Alarms, reminders, music.
    - A morning playlist that cues energy.
    - A bedtime meditation track that cues sleep.

3. **Temporal** - time-based cues.
    - Every morning, stretch for two minutes.
    - After lunch/dinner, walk for ten.
    - Before bed, breathe deeply.
4. **Social** - who you're around.
    - Tell someone your goal.
    - Join a group or a class.
    - Have a walking buddy or accountability partner.

When you align triggers with the habits you're trying to build, the results follow naturally.

Example - Designing Hydration, Not Hoping for It

Let's say hydration is your weak point. It's not enough to vaguely promise, *"I'll drink more water."* That's not a system, that's a wish.

Instead:
- Set an alarm every hour.
- Use a water bottle with measurements.
- Keep water within arm's reach everywhere you sit.

Now hydration is no longer about remembering, your being reminded by your environment. That's designing for success.

Hydration is one of the simplest but most overlooked pillars of regeneration. Most people either don't drink enough or over-complicate it. They get lost in debates about whether it should be two litres, three litres, or eight glasses.

Here's the truth: **there is no magic number.** The right amount depends on your body, your size, your activity, your environment. What matters is not litres but *measurement*.

This is the rule of thumb I give patients:
Every time you have a full drink, you should go to the toilet. When you go to the toilet, it should be clear enough so that you know you're hydrated.

If you're not, you're not drinking enough. Simple as that.

Don't get hung up on numbers, instead focus on the outcome. Use the 5-star weekly urine output chart (from the Time chapter, page 321).

This way hydration is no longer about willpower. It's about environment, awareness and outcome.

Example - Designing Movement Into the Day

Perhaps movement is your issue. For many people, the idea of the gym is intimidating, unrealistic, time consuming or just unappealing and that's fine. You don't need a gym to regenerate. In fact, most of my patients don't stick with gyms, because it's not designed into their lives, it's an add-on, an appointment, an extra burden.

What you need is movement woven into the rhythm of your day.

Consider movement as a continuous force in all your activities. The power of daily habits outweighs the effect of a sporadic, high-intensity workout. Your body prefers a consistent rhythm over a jarring surprise.

Here are some examples:
- Stand up while you're on calls.
- Stretch or do squats while waiting for the microwave.
- Park further from the supermarket door.
- Walk the long way back from the bathroom.

Habits

- Do ten calf raises while brushing your teeth.
- Carry shopping bags evenly to balance your posture.

None of these look like "exercise", but that's the point. They don't require gym clothes, equipment, or an hour carved out of your diary. They require nothing more than awareness and a small decision in the moment.

You've already seen C.R.A.F.T. in the Physics chapter: **C**ontrol, **R**epeatability, **A**symmetry, **F**low, **T**wist. That framework isn't just for clinics or athletes. It's a reminder that the way you move, every day, matters.

When you're designing for success, don't just think about whether you're moving but how. Are you in control, or are you powering through with sloppy form? Are you repeating good mechanics, or building bad ones? Are you twisting awkwardly or sitting in ways that unbalance you?

Designing smarter movement isn't about adding more hours. It's about applying the same principles to your ordinary day. C.R.A.F.T. keeps the quality high and it stops you rehearsing poor mechanics. It reminds you that regeneration isn't about smashing workouts; it's about weaving quality movement into the structure of life.

Why this matters

Movement is medicine. It keeps joints lubricated, muscles activated, blood flowing and the nervous system switched on. A sedentary body switches off, circulation slows, muscles waste, stiffness creeps in and injuries take longer to heal. The number one mistake people make is assuming that unless they're sweating in lycra, it doesn't count.

Let's face it, your body doesn't care about your membership card. It cares about load, rhythm and use. Muscles that are used, even lightly, stay alive, joints that are moved regularly stay mobile and tendons that are loaded adapt and strengthen.

This is why I tell patients: *don't aim for "workouts", aim for daily deposits into the movement bank.* Small, regular credits compound faster than occasional lump sums.

The 1% Rule

Think about marginal gains. If you can increase your daily movement by even 1%, one extra flight of stairs (provided your knees are ok), one extra stand-up break or one short walk, the compounding effect over weeks and months is enormous.

- An extra 500 steps per day adds up to 3,500 steps a week; that's like walking roughly a marathon every four months, without noticing.
- Standing for 2 minutes every hour adds 16 minutes of circulation a day, nearly 2 hours a week, over 100 hours a year.
- Ten calf raises twice a day equals over 7,000 in a year; that's enough to change your ankle strength and balance permanently.

None of that requires a gym, it requires thought.
The body doesn't respond best to shock, it responds best to rhythm. That's why the 1% rule works so powerfully: you don't overhaul everything in one day; you make tiny changes for longer periods.

The compounding effect of rhythm beats the short-lived drama of intensity every time. A gym session once a week might leave you sore, but it won't build resilience. Consistent micro-movements, threaded into your day, rewire your body's baseline.

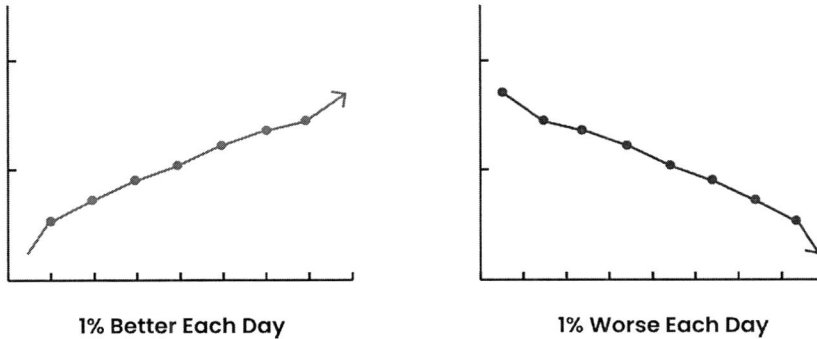

1% Better Each Day   1% Worse Each Day

Building It In

Here's the trick: don't treat movement as an optional add-on. Treat it like brushing your teeth, it happens every day, multiple times, without a debate. That's what designing movement into your day looks like.

Start by asking yourself: *where are my "dead zones", the times I'm waiting, scrolling, or sitting unnecessarily?* Turn those dead zones into movement opportunities.

Waiting for the kids at school – walk laps around the car park. Sat on the sofa streaming – sit on an exercise ball or hold a tin in each hand and do some arm exercises while watching.

Dead time becomes alive time.

Movement as Identity

The best exercise is the one you keep doing, and most people stick with the movement that fits naturally into their day and feels like life rather than a workout.

When you design movement into your day, you stop thinking of yourself as "someone who needs to exercise". You become "someone who moves". That identity shift is where you want to be.

Flow & Focus

Designing success isn't only about the body, it's about the mind. Focus is a habit too.

There are three keys I teach patients and professionals:
1. **Design your environment**: cluttered places create cluttered thoughts. Clear your space and your mind clears with it.
2. **Block your time**: focus works like a muscle. Set aside 30–60 minutes for one task, silence notifications and give it your full attention.
3. **Manage your energy**: don't expect peak focus at midnight if your natural rhythm is in the morning. Align hard tasks with high energy, light tasks with low energy.

Do this and you create flow: that state where work feels effortless, time disappears and performance peaks. Flow doesn't come by accident, it comes by design.

It might seem obvious reading it here, but if you stop and think about what holds you back, it's likely to be time, environment or energy.

Plan for Failure, Not Motivation

Here's the brutal truth: motivation is short-lived. It's exciting on day one, maybe day two but by day five, motivation has waned if not already packed up. Life is messy, stress shows up, sleep suffers, the kids get sick and work piles up and suddenly that "new you" feels like a distant dream.

Many people imagine with the right incentive, they'll always feel inspired, but success doesn't come from motivation. It comes from planning.

One of my favourite sayings is: ***"Fail to plan, plan to fail."***

That's not just about having a perfect schedule or a colour-coded diary. It's about knowing that life will throw you off course and having a plan for what happens when it does, because you *will* fail, you *will* get derailed and that's not weakness, that's human.

As I often remind patients: *we take action by emotion.* How we feel creates our thoughts and our thoughts create our actions. If you're tired, stressed, or overwhelmed, you won't feel like doing the good thing, so, if you rely on motivation alone, you'll do nothing.

That's why designing for failure matters.

The Environment Equation

So how do you do it? You create an environment that nudges you towards health even on the worst days.
- If the biscuit tin is hidden on the top shelf, you'll consider what you're doing when you have to physically reach for it and be more likely to choose something healthier.
- If your calendar has a blocked-out 15 minutes, it becomes protected space to breathe or stretch.
- If your TV remote lives on the bookshelf next to a resistance band, you're more likely to pick both up together.

Environment drives emotion. Emotion drives thought. Thought drives action. Set the tone, set the scene and you've already won half the battle.

Your Fallback Plan

Motivation says: "I'll do an hour at the gym."
Design says: "What's my five-minute version of this habit?"

That's your fallback.

On the day you can't be bothered, what will you do instead?
- If you can't face a run, walk around the block.
- If you're too busy for meditation, take three deep breaths.
- If you missed your workout, stretch for two minutes.

These are not trivial. They're persistence in action. They keep the identity alive: *we still do this.*

Persistent and Consistent

I always come back to two words: **persistent and consistent.**

Persistence means you don't quit when it gets hard.

Consistency means you keep showing up, even in small ways.

It doesn't matter if your action is reduced or imperfect. What matters is that you act. Because every small action reinforces the loop: I am someone who regenerates.

Plan for Reset

Finally, plan the reset. Don't just accept that you'll fail, expect it and decide now how you'll respond.

The biggest mistake people make is beating themselves up. They treat one missed day as a disaster and that guilt becomes the excuse to give up altogether. Failure isn't final; it's feedback. Missing a habit doesn't mean you've blown it; it means you've discovered a weak point in your system. The worst thing you can do is to treat one puncture as a reason to slash the other three tyres.

Behavioural science backs this up. Carol Dweck's research on growth mindset shows that people who see setbacks as information, not condemnation, are the ones who improve.

The rule is: stumble, then reset fast. Don't wait until Monday, don't wait for "when life calms down". Reset now. Shrink the habit if you must, from a walk to a stretch, from a stretch to a breath but get back in the loop. That's how persistence gets built, not in the days when everything's easy but in the moments you refuse to let failure define you.

Say you miss your exercise session; that doesn't mean you have to give up and go back to doing nothing. Fail does not equal stop. It just means you pick up again tomorrow, or even later the same day if you can.

Instead, reset with perspective. Ask yourself: why did I fall off? What was missing from my environment, my plan, or my energy? Learn from it. Adjust. Then start again.

One missed day isn't failure. The only failure is refusing to get back on track.

If you live with chronic pain, you will miss days. That's the reality of working with a body that demands more care. The answer isn't to push through recklessly but to adjust intelligently. On bad days, shrink the habit: pain is a signal, not a stop sign.

So, plan your reset like this:
1. Acknowledge it without guilt. Everyone falls.
2. Learn from it. What tripped you up?
3. Restart quickly. Don't wait for Monday, or next month. Start now.

That's how you stop a stumble becoming a collapse. That's how persistence gets built.

The Five-Minute Habit Arsenal

Here's a list I can recommend, the "five-minute arsenal". These are things you can do even on your worst day:
- 10 reps of an exercise while the kettle boils.
- 2 minutes of deep breathing.
- Lie on the floor with your legs up the wall.
- Listen to a funny podcast.
- Drink a glass of water.
- Step outside and feel the sun on your face.
- Write one line of gratitude.
- 30 seconds of laughing out loud.

On a bad day, just choose one. That's all it takes.

You see, here's the thing: the day you feel like doing nothing is the most important day to do something. Even a small something. It keeps the habit alive. It tells your brain: *we still do this.*

The Psychology of Persistence

Every small action you take sends a signal to your body and mind about who you are and what you value.

Roll your shoulders and open your chest when you stand up from your desk → you're reinforcing that posture is part of performance.

Switch off screens an hour before bed → you're showing you protect your circadian rhythm.

Prep a healthy lunch instead of grabbing fast food → you're reinforcing that you fuel, not just feed.

Journal one line of gratitude → you're proving you invest in your mental wellbeing.

Do balance work while brushing teeth → you're showing you care about mobility as you age.

No single action defines you, but the repetition builds identity. Over time, those signals accumulate until they become automatic – part of who you are.

This is why I say: stop aiming for perfection. Build the identity by repeating the action.

The Goal

Most people fail not because they're incapable but because they didn't plan for the moment they'd want to quit.

Designing for success isn't about copying someone else's system. It's about creating one that works for you.
- Some people thrive on structure whilst others rebel against it.

- Some need music to focus, others need silence.
- Some love tech, others prefer pen and paper.

There's no universal blueprint. The only truth is this: if it's not personal, it won't last.

So, Experiment – Adjust – Reflect – Notice - what sticks and what doesn't.

This is the **EARN principle**, because every habit, every bit of progress, has to be earned.
- **Experiment** – try different approaches until you find what fits.
- **Adjust** – when it doesn't stick, change the design, not the goal.
- **Reflect** – step back and ask what's working and what isn't.
- **Notice** – pay attention to the small wins, because they show you where to build next.

The truth is, no system works out of the box. You earn your success by shaping it until it fits your life.

If you find yourself dropping a habit, that's not proof you're weak, it's proof that the design didn't quite fit. Tweak or adapt it. Sometimes the smallest change makes the biggest difference: shifting the time of day, changing the trigger, or lowering the barrier to entry.

From Effort to Identity

The final piece of designing for success is understanding how habits move from effort to ease. At the beginning, every action feels deliberate. It takes energy. You're fighting against old defaults, that's normal.

However, if you stay with it, the balance shifts. What once felt awkward starts to feel natural. What once required discipline starts to feel like part of who you are.

That's not luck or willpower; that's biology adapting to the signals you keep giving it. Repetition strengthens the pathways in your brain until the new pattern becomes the default. This is why bad habits hold on so tightly and why building good ones takes patience. You are literally re-engineering yourself.

This is why I always come back to two words: *persistent and consistent.*
- Persistence is refusing to quit when you miss.
- Consistency is showing up often enough to let the wiring take hold.

Put those together and you create momentum that doesn't rely on inspiration.

Identity in Motion

The real shift isn't when you tick off a habit on a checklist. It's when you stop seeing regeneration as something you "do" and start seeing it as something you *are*.

Here's the key: you don't have to embody all of regeneration at once. That's not realistic and it's not the point.

Start by choosing one small action from one pillar. Maybe it's physics – doing a daily stretch. Maybe it's chemistry – cutting out one processed snack, just one and nail that. Let it become part of the norm for you, so much so that you don't even consider it.

Once that's in place, you then layer. Add one, then another. Over time, the identity grows stronger because each action reinforces it. You're no longer "someone trying to change". You're the person who regenerates, not perfectly, not completely but consistently, piece by piece.

Regeneration is the layering of micro activities that hold together over time.

Identity & Four Pillars

Identity isn't built in one domain. True regeneration comes when your habits stretch across the four pillars:
- **Physics:** "I am someone who moves with awareness. I respect posture, mechanics and the strength and stability of my frame."
- **Chemistry:** "I am someone who pays attention to what goes in, what breaks down and what comes out. I fuel with nutrition, balance my chemistry and don't fight my body with the wrong inputs."
- **Biology:** "I am someone who honours my internal rhythms. I care for my gut, my nervous system, my sleep and the living forest that is my body."

- **Time:** "I am someone who respects the timelines of healing. I protect recovery, monitor progress and invest today so that future decades are strong."

When these pillars line up, identity stops being an aspiration and becomes the way you live.

Regen PhD: a Toolkit designed for regeneration

The Pod

Throughout this book, you've seen the four pillars of regeneration. Each one matters in its own right but in real life, they never stand alone, they are interdependent. Move and you're in physics straight away but you're also drawing on chemistry (ATP, electrolytes, hormones) and loading tissues that biology must repair. Change what you eat and you're altering chemistry first, which then reshapes biology (microbiome, inflammation, hormones) and ultimately changes how you move. Recovery sits in biology, but it only works when you give it time.

That interdependence is exactly why I designed the Regen PhD Pod. Regeneration doesn't happen in fragments; it happens when the pillars meet.

In physics, we looked at force and function. The pod supports this by easing posture, symmetry and mobility with vibration, traction and heat.

In chemistry, we explored the invisible war of nutrition, hormones and inflammation. The pod amplifies circulation, reduces inflammation and strengthens the internal environment so chemistry works with you rather than against you.

In biology, we saw the body as a forest. The pod works here too, with inputs that align with circadian cycles, neurological patterns and the subtle rhythms of recovery.

In time, we faced the reality that biology can't be rushed, but time can be used better. The pod helps compress wasted time, reducing decline that comes from delay, injury or inaction. It doesn't replace months of work, but it prevents months of damage.

The problem for most people is a scattered approach. You see a physio for movement, travel across town for a sauna or red light therapy session. You've got supplements in one cupboard and a book on breathing practices gathering dust. The effort is fragmented and so the results are fragmented.

The pod was designed to end this. It brings the essentials into one place, one rhythm, one system, so regeneration isn't a list of errands but a single integrated experience.

Not everyone can build habits from scratch. Some people are too busy, too stressed, too overwhelmed and that's exactly why I built the pod, as a foundation. It's not a substitute for good habits but it's a shortcut to get started. If you don't yet have the time or structure to establish routines, the pod gives you a rhythm to build from.

However, nothing works with one session. Consistency and persistency are non-negotiable. That's why pod use is structured: six sessions minimum, once or twice a week. That rhythm matters. With repeated use, the body adapts, energy builds, sleep improves and the system begins to reset.

There are other tools out there: red light therapy, saunas, cold immersion. They all have value but only if you do them consistently. The principle behind the pod is different. It doesn't rely on you piecing those things together one by one, rather it combines proven accelerators and delivers them in harmony, a supercharge, not a slow drip.

The pod, the protocols and the tools, they don't do the work for you. They preserve, protect and accelerate, giving you the momentum to build the habits that matter. They don't replace regeneration, they reinforce it.

That's what makes the pod different: a system, a bridge between the four pillars, built so you can experience regeneration in real time.

Protocols: The Rhythm

Nothing in regeneration works as a one-off. You can't eat one salad and call yourself healthy or do one workout and expect strength. The same goes for the pod.

That's why the protocols are structured over a minimum of six sessions, once or twice weekly.

One session might feel good and you may notice a lift in energy, better sleep, even less pain, but it won't last. The body needs repetition to lock in the benefits. Just like the six-day ignition and six-week embedding we've already talked about with habits, the pod requires rhythm to work.

Each pod session delivers the same five elements of energy in a consistent pattern, and that's what creates the shift:
- **Heat** to open vessels and prime tissue
- **Light** to stimulate mitochondria
- **Sound** to guide your nervous system into regulation
- **Vibration** to mobilise lymph and release tension
- **Magnetic input** to restore electrical balance

One session is a spark, six sessions create a flame. Keep going and the fire sustains itself.

Here's why:
- **Adaptation takes time.** Muscles, nerves and connective tissues respond to repeated signals, not isolated ones.
- **Systems need reinforcement.** Circulation, sleep cycles and hormonal balance reset gradually, not instantly.
- **Habits need anchors.** A weekly pod session isn't just therapy; it's a reminder, a cue to live in alignment with the four pillars the rest of the week.
- **Energy is layered.** The pod works with the five elements of energy you've already met in this book: heat, light, vibration, sound and magnetic input, and those only create real change when they're delivered consistently, not sporadically.

Without rhythm, even the best technology is wasted, yet with rhythm, the benefits compound. Energy builds instead of draining, sleep deepens instead of breaking and pain lessens instead of escalating.

This is why I don't offer the pod as a "drop-in quick fix". That's like going to the gym once and judging exercise a failure. The pod is a tool for persistence, and persistence only shows its power over time.

Protocols: The Accelerators

As I've shown you, the pod isn't built around one therapy. It's built around layers. Each accelerator plays its part, but the real power comes when they're combined in sequence.
- **Negative ions** help reset your internal balance, calming the nervous system.
- **Graphene far-infrared heat** penetrates deep into the muscles, easing tightness and helping the whole body relax from the inside out.
- **Extremity far-infrared** directs circulation into the legs and feet, the areas most prone to sluggish flow.
- **Near-infrared light** charges the mitochondria, fuelling the cells for repair and resilience.
- **Bio-harmonic vibration** promotes circulation and fluid movement, like a gentle massage for the whole system.
- **Rotating electromagnetic fields** stir biology at a cellular level, boosting circulation and cellular vitality.
- **Jade thermal base** grounds and stabilises the session, holding warmth and balance.
- **Terahertz waveform** adds a frontier frequency, subtle but exciting in its early regenerative potential.

On their own, each of these has value importantly, together, they work in harmony. It's the difference between hearing instruments tune up individually and listening to an orchestra play in sync.

The accelerators aren't there to replace your habits, they're there to amplify them. To give your biology a push so that your efforts outside the pod take root more quickly and hold more firmly.

That's why I call it a supercharge, because it compresses what works slowly on its own into a shorter, more powerful experience.

Protocols: EMS and TENS

Separate from the Pod, but essential to the wider regenerative system, are the EMS and TENS protocols I developed. These are not add-ons or shortcuts. They exist to protect momentum at moments when the body is most vulnerable to loss.

Electrical Muscle Stimulation (EMS) is about preservation, not performance. Its role is to keep muscle tissue awake when normal signals are disrupted. After injury or surgery, the brain often down-regulates muscle activation to protect the area. The problem is that protection quickly turns into shutdown. Within days, muscle fibres begin to switch off. Within weeks, measurable muscle loss follows.

In some cases, as much as 30 percent of muscle mass can be lost in the first two weeks after surgery if the muscle is left unstimulated. That loss is not just cosmetic. It reduces joint stability, slows rehabilitation, alters movement patterns and places additional stress on surrounding structures. Once that decline sets in, recovery becomes longer, harder and less predictable.

EMS interrupts this cascade. By providing an external electrical signal, it reminds the muscle how to contract even when voluntary movement is limited or inhibited. Fibres continue to fire. Blood flow is maintained. Neuromuscular pathways stay engaged. Instead of restarting from zero weeks later, the system remains primed for recovery.

TENS works differently but just as strategically. Rather than contracting muscle, it targets the nervous system. Pain is not simply a sensation; it is a signal that shapes behaviour. When pain dominates, people stop moving, sleep poorly and hold tension in protective patterns. That environment is hostile to regeneration.

TENS reduces pain signalling by interrupting the transmission of nociceptive input to the brain. In simple terms, it quietens the noise. That quiet matters. When pain is reduced, sleep improves. When sleep improves, hormone balance stabilises. When movement feels safer, people begin to re-engage with normal activity rather than guarding and avoiding.

Used together, EMS and TENS create a powerful support structure. EMS preserves muscle integrity and readiness. TENS lowers the barriers that pain creates. Circulation improves. Movement becomes possible earlier. The nervous system stops bracing and starts recalibrating.

When these protocols are combined with Pod work, the effect is cumulative. Muscle is protected. Pain is managed. Tissue receives better blood flow and oxygenation. The body is held in a state where regeneration is more likely to occur and less likely to be derailed by shutdown, fear or fatigue.

This is the logic of habits in regeneration. Small, consistent inputs applied at the right time prevent large losses later. EMS and TENS are not about doing more. They are about stopping the system from slipping backwards while recovery is still unfolding.

Regeneration rarely fails because people do too little, it fails because the body loses ground quietly while waiting. These protocols exist to make sure that waiting does not become wasting.

Other Regen Developments

The pod is only one part of the bigger picture. My work has always been about taking regeneration out of theory and putting it into people's lives, especially in the areas medicine tends to overlook. That's why I've been developing new tools and new clinics, because these are the gaps I see every day in my patients, the places where people are left to struggle in silence.

Take the Regen PhD Chair. People suffering tend to be uncomfortable talking about bladder weakness, pelvic pain or sexual health. Yet these issues affect millions and they undermine confidence, mobility and quality of life. The chair was built to bring regeneration right to the centre of the body: the pelvic floor. Using advanced stimulation, it helps retrain and restore the muscles that hold everything else together. When the core is compromised, it doesn't just affect movement, it affects how you feel about yourself, so the chair gives people a way back.

The Lee Liquid Cartilage™ Procedure (LLC Protocol)

One of the most important projects I have taken from concept to clinic is the Lee Liquid Cartilage Procedure™. It exists for one reason: cartilage can heal, but only when the conditions are right.

The problem has never been the biology but the conditions. Cartilage needs structure, signalling, stability, and time. When any one of those is missing, repair fails.

The LLC Protocol was designed to restore this framework.

Instead of removing damaged tissue and hoping for the best, this approach creates a scaffold inside the joint that allows your own cells to rebuild. Your biology does the work; the procedure provides the framework. Surgery becomes a starting point, not the solution.

What matters just as much as the operation is what follows. Early muscle activation, carefully staged loading, and nutritional support turn repair into function. This is regeneration by design in practice: physics to manage load, chemistry to support tissue formation, biology to guide healing, and time respected rather than rushed.

Every joint, every injury, and every person is different. That is why this is not a fixed recipe. It is a framework that adapts to the individual. When engineering and biology are aligned properly, the body does what it has always been capable of doing.

You can find out more about the process in depth on my website.

How It Works

The procedure uses a collagen hydrogel scaffold called ChondroFiller™. It sets inside the joint, forming a 3D structure for new cartilage cells to grow into. Into that scaffold, I add your own biological materials such as platelet-rich plasma (PRP), platelet-rich fibrin (PRF) and, in selected cases, medicinal signalling cells (MSCs) from bone marrow or fat.

To stabilise and support the repair, I use tranexamic acid (TXA) to protect the fibrin clots and IV vitamins to help the collagen form stronger cross-links. Then comes the part most people overlook, the recovery system. Early muscle activation through EMS, carefully staged loading and tailored nutrition turn the initial repair into lasting function.

This is what I mean by Regeneration by Design in Action: balancing physics, chemistry and biology so the body can rebuild from within.

Regenerating Through Hormonal Change

One of the areas I've been putting more energy into is menopause and andropause. These transitions affect the whole system: bone density, muscle strength, cardiovascular health, sleep, cognition and mood. They change how your body recovers and adapts.

Too often, people are given a prescription and told to carry on but as you now know, hormones don't work in isolation, they affect movement, metabolism and mental health. If we only medicate, we miss the chance to support the whole person.

That's why I've brought together colleagues from medicine, physiotherapy, rehabilitation and movement training. Together, we're looking at these transitions as opportunities for recalibration. With the right assessments, supplements and targeted therapies, this stage can be the point where you reinforce your system, not watch it break down. We're now offering clinics and wellness consultations; you can find out more here: https://menopause.regenphd.com

Why do I push so hard on this - because regeneration isn't optional. If you lose pelvic strength, it changes your independence. If you ignore menopause, you risk decades of preventable decline and if you guess at supplements, you waste time and money while your body pays the price. This is central to your overall wellness.

Genetic Insights and Regeneration

Genetic and epigenetic analysis are the next frontiers in regeneration. Your DNA doesn't dictate your destiny, but it does reveal your tendencies. When you understand those tendencies, you can stop relying on guesswork and start making choices that align with your biology.

This is how it connects to the four pillars:
- **Physics**: Your genes can influence muscle fibre type, joint structure and recovery speed. If we know you're predisposed to slower recovery, we build your movement plan differently.
- **Chemistry**: Genetic markers affect how you metabolise nutrients, respond to certain foods and manage inflammation. Tailoring diet and supplements becomes more precise.

- **Biology**: Hormonal balance, sleep patterns and stress responses are all affected by your genetic profile. Epigenetics then shows how lifestyle switches those systems on or off.
- **Time**: Epigenetic testing reveals biological age; not how many years you've lived but how well your cells are functioning. It tells us if you're ageing faster or slower than your birth certificate suggests.

By layering these insights on top of clinical practice, we move from a general programme to a personalised map. The DNA12 health programme I've developed takes this further by running monthly checks across areas like cardiac risk, fatigue, hormone balance and organ health. Instead of snapshots, we build a moving picture of your health. That way, we can adapt your regeneration plan in real time.

This is about clarity, showing you where you're strong, where you're vulnerable and how your habits are shaping your biology today.

The pod and the protocols give you a starting point, the DNA and epigenetic testing give you a map, then the real future of regeneration goes even further. My work now is focused on creating systems that don't just give you feedback every few months but live dashboards of your health, motion analysis, biology, chemistry and time all feeding into one model.

What's Next for Regeneration

So where do we go from here?

The future isn't about adding more isolated tools it's about integration. It's about building systems that bring everything together, so you get a complete, living picture of your health.

This is the direction my work is taking now: bringing physics, chemistry, biology and time into one model. Not a glimpse, a blood test every six months or a scan once a year but a live system that reflects who you are right now and where you're heading.

The Digital Twin

The idea is simple but powerful: a *digital twin*. A model of you that runs alongside you, built from your data, your movement patterns, your blood markers, hormone levels, sleep cycles, DNA and epigenetics. Every piece of information we can gather feeds into this model. The more data we put in, the clearer the picture becomes.

Why does this matter?

A digital twin is exactly that: a living record of you, a model that reflects not just where you are now but how you're changing over time. That alone is powerful. It means we can spot a decline early, correct the course before it becomes a crisis and personalise interventions to the individual rather than the average.

The twin isn't just about tracking forwards, it's about preserving backwards. Imagine this: at 55, we capture your biology when it's strong, resilient and stable. Then, at 60, if something starts to fail, we don't just treat the symptoms, we look back at the 55-year-old version of you and we ask: how do we restore those cells, that function, that resilience?

That's the potential. Not just slowing decline but rewinding it. Using the record of your younger self as a blueprint for repair.

We're not there yet but the foundations are being laid and the reason I push this forward is simple: if we wait until you're unwell, the clock has already run down. If we build the record now, we have the baseline to work from later. It's not just prevention; it's preservation.

That's the future of regeneration. A health record that isn't just paperwork, it's you, stored, protected and ready to guide both today's decisions and tomorrow's breakthroughs.

Habits

The AI Dashboard

This is where it gets really exciting. The benefit of AI isn't just spotting patterns in today's data, it's preserving you at your best, so we've got a blueprint to return to when life throws something at you.

Take an injury, for instance. Right now, most rehab starts from the point of damage: we test where you are after the event and then build a plan from there, however, if I already have your digital twin: the exact way your hip rotated, how your knee tracked, the balance of your stride, the firing order of your muscles, then rehab isn't guesswork anymore. It's precision engineering. I don't just say, "let's strengthen this leg", I can say, "this is how your body moved before and this is the roadmap to get you back there."

Now imagine major surgery. Today, you wake up in recovery and we monitor your vitals from scratch. Yet what if we already know your baseline: your heart variability, sleep rhythms, hormone responses, even your joint stability? With that data banked, we can rebuild you to your normal, not some generic average. That changes everything.

Here's where it really blows my mind – ageing. If I've got your cellular and motion data at 60 and at 70 something slips – arthritis, fatigue, a loss of coordination – then I can look back at that "60 version" and ask, how do we coax you back there? Maybe not entirely but enough to restore function and to reset the system. That's regeneration in its purest form: not just slowing decline but rewinding towards a younger state of health.

This is why I get so fired up about the digital twin. It's not science fiction - it's science applied with intelligence. We already have the tech, MRI, motion analysis, AI pattern recognition. We just need to connect the dots and when we do, recovery stops being trial-and-error, it becomes targeted, personal and frankly, a bit revolutionary.

From Reaction to Design

For too long, medicine has been built on reaction: wait for symptoms, then treat. The future I'm describing is about design: measure early, act early, adapt often. It's about replacing crisis management with continuous support.

The cool thing is that the tools are already here: motion analysis, pods, EMS, DNA testing, epigenetics and AI dashboards. The work now is to link them, refine them and make them accessible.

That's what drives me. My energy goes into designing systems that people can rely on, systems that strengthen, restore and protect. Everything I create is about helping people live not just longer but stronger, with more vitality, more clarity and more control over their health. That's the real goal: not adding years to life but adding life to years.

Ownership and Empowerment

Let me be clear – this isn't just for doctors; the point of a digital twin isn't to make medicine more complicated. It's to give *you* ownership, because when you can see your own trajectory, in black and white, in numbers and visuals, you don't have to take it on faith. You know where you are, what's working and you can decide what to change.

That's the empowerment people are craving. Too many patients come to me feeling lost in the system, passed from one specialist to another, collecting reports they don't understand. A digital twin changes that, it puts everything in one place and lets you see the forest as well as the trees.

From Individuals to Humanity

But there's another layer to this vision. The digital twin isn't just about one person at a time. Imagine millions of twins, millions of people feeding data into a global system. With consent and privacy protected, the collective insights could transform what we know about human health.

Patterns of disease could be spotted years earlier, effective protocols could be refined faster. Preventive strategies could be tested and scaled globally, instead of waiting for decades of research, we'd have real-time evidence from real lives.

That's the bigger picture - Regeneration at scale.

The Live Forever Movement

I call this the Live Forever Movement. Not because I think we'll ever stop ageing altogether but because I know we can live younger for longer and pass on the systems that make it possible.

For you, that means strength, clarity and energy that doesn't run out just because you've reached a certain age. For humanity, it means that the work we're doing now, the measurements, the data, the systems, becomes the foundation for the next generation. They don't start from zero. They start from where we leave off.

That's the legacy. If Newton said he stood on the shoulders of giants, then we must decide to be those shoulders. Every step you take, every piece of data we store, every tool we refine, becomes part of that future.

This is how I see the next era of medicine: not waiting for symptoms and reacting but designing regeneration in advance. Measure early. Act early. Adapt continuously. Use the tools we already have: pods, motion analysis, EMS, DNA mapping, epigenetics, AI; not in isolation but as a living system that grows stronger the longer you use it.

That's what I mean by living forever. Not adding years for the sake of it but making the years you have worth more. Not letting decline be the default but choosing design instead.

As for living forever in the truest sense? Well… that's for the next book.

Acknowledgements

I would like to thank my parents, Panny and Aaron, for their unwavering support throughout my education and professional journey. Their belief in learning, perseverance, and long-term thinking created the foundation on which everything else has been built.

To my brother Philip, and his family — thank you for your continued encouragement and for standing beside me as ideas became reality. From education to innovation, and now in building Regen PhD, your support has mattered deeply.

I would also like to thank my father-in-law, David, for his support, steadiness, and presence within our family. That support — often quiet and unspoken — has been sincerely appreciated.

I would also like to acknowledge my sister-in-law, Lowri, for her help, care, and support to our family over the years. These contributions, often given without expectation or recognition, have been genuinely appreciated.

I wish to express my deepest gratitude to Mr Leonidas Vachtsevanos, a close friend of over twenty-five years. His support

Acknowledgements

during my darkest hours — professionally, mentally, and academically — was unwavering. His belief, perspective, and loyalty carried me through moments that would otherwise have been insurmountable. This journey would not have been possible without him.

I am grateful to my international colleagues and friends who share a common philosophy: that staying young, staying strong, and extending human capability is not about fear of ageing, but about responsibility to future generations.

In particular, I would like to thank:
- Professor Cristiano Paggetti (Orthokey), for sharing the vision behind MAI Motion and believing that objective movement intelligence is central to the future of musculoskeletal health.
- Dr Yan Wen, whose scientific depth and persistence made on MRI possible, transforming imaging into meaningful, quantitative insight.
- Dr Tanvi Verma, for her leadership, resilience, and commitment in sustaining and advancing the research department.
- Professor Feza Korkusuz, a valued colleague and friend, for exploring the biochemical and biological dimensions of regeneration with me, and for deepening our understanding of regenerative therapies at a cellular and molecular level.
- Sally Edwards, for her unwavering support and for ensuring that patients are always cared for with professionalism, dignity, and humanity.
- Helen Morris, our physiotherapist, for continually pushing the boundaries of rehabilitation and

reminding us that regeneration is expressed through movement and function, not procedures alone.
- Alan del Rosario and Rhoderick Panganiban, for making regenerative surgery possible in practice and for their essential role in data collection, without which learning, refinement, and progress would not exist.

Finally, I thank the patients.

You remind us that regeneration is not about living forever in years alone — it is about staying capable, strong, and purposeful. When strength, knowledge, and kindness are passed on, something far greater than biology endures.

Author Bio

Professor Paul Lee is a Consultant Orthopaedic Surgeon, Medical Engineer, and the author of *Practical Regeneration*.

He specialises in joint preservation, regenerative medicine and movement health, with a strong focus on prevention, early intervention and long-term function.

He holds a PhD in Medical Engineering, has postgraduate training in sports and regenerative medicine, and works at the intersection of clinical practice, biomechanics and applied science.

He is an Honorary Professor of Sports Medicine at the University of Lincoln and served as Visiting Professor of Medical Engineering at the University of Chester until 2025.

Alongside his clinical work, he is actively involved in research, innovation and education aimed at improving health literacy and supporting more sustainable approaches to healthcare.

His work translates complex medical and engineering principles into clear, practical frameworks that empower people to move better, make confident decisions and age with greater strength and resilience.

Regeneration made simple.

You can find out more about Professor Lee and the Regen PhD Pod at:

Other Books by Professor Paul Lee

Regeneration by Design - The Science of Superhuman Ageing - published by ReThink Press 2024

Musculoskeletal Regeneration Medicine - Published by Springer Cham 2025

Coming Soon

Regen Made Simple

Further Reading

Core Scientific Foundations
(Regenerative medicine, biology, neuroscience, endocrinology)

de Grey, A., & Rae, M. (2007). *Ending Aging: The rejuvenation breakthroughs that could reverse human aging in our lifetime.* New York: St Martin's Press.

Newson, L. (2024) *The Definitive Guide to the Perimenopause and Menopause.* London. Yellow Kite

Sapolsky, R. M. (2004). *Why Zebras Don't Get Ulcers* (3rd ed.). New York: Holt Paperbacks.

Sapolsky, R. M. (2017). *Behave: The biology of humans at our best and worst.* London: Penguin Press.

Sinclair, D. A., & LaPlante, M. (2019). *Lifespan: Why we age and why we don't have to.* London: HarperCollins.

van der Kolk, B. (2014). *The Body Keeps the Score: Brain, mind and body in the healing of trauma.* London: Penguin Books.

Walker, M. (2017). *Why We Sleep: Unlocking the power of sleep and dreams.* London: Allen Lane.

Movement, Physics and Biomechanics
(Gait analysis, load, MAI-Motion foundations)

Blakeslee, S., & Blakeslee, M. (2007). *The Body Has a Mind of Its Own: How body maps in your brain help you do almost everything better.* New York: Random House.

Bowman, K. (2014). *Move Your DNA: Restore your health through natural movement.* Propriometrics Press.

Kirtley, C. (2006). *Clinical Gait Analysis: Theory and practice.* Edinburgh: Churchill Livingstone.

Starrett, K., & Cordoza, G. (2015). *Becoming a Supple Leopard.* San Francisco: Victory Belt Publishing.

Energy and Electromagnetic Therapies
(Photobiomodulation, PEMF, vibration)

Becker, R. O., & Selden, G. (1985). *The Body Electric: Electromagnetism and the foundation of life.* New York: William Morrow.

Oschman, J. L. (2015). *Energy Medicine: The scientific basis.* Edinburgh: Churchill Livingstone.

Systems, Time and Preventative Health
Attia, P., & Gifford, B. (2023). *Outlive: The science and art of longevity.* London: Harmony.

Clear, J. (2018). *Atomic Habits.* London: Random House Business.

Epstein, D. (2019). *Range: Why generalists triumph in a specialised world.* London: Pan Macmillan.

Topol, E. (2019). *Deep Medicine: How artificial intelligence can make healthcare human again.* London: Basic Books.

Historical and Foundational Texts Referenced
(Contextual lineage, not clinical instruction)

Aurelius, M. (c. 170 CE). *Meditations.* Various modern translations.

Hippocrates. (c. 400 BCE). *Hippocratic Corpus.* Translated collections.

Laozi. (c. 6th century BCE). *Tao Te Ching.* Various modern translations.

Sun Tzu. (c. 5th century BCE). *The Art of War.* Various modern translations.

Unschuld, P. U. (Trans.). (2016). *The Yellow Emperor's Classic of Medicine.* Berkeley: University of California Press.